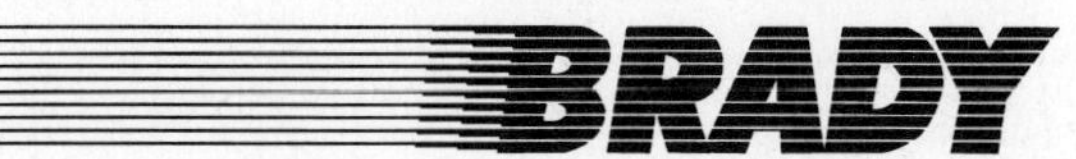

Workbook

From Nursing Assistant to Clinical Care Associate

Carole Miele
Teresa England

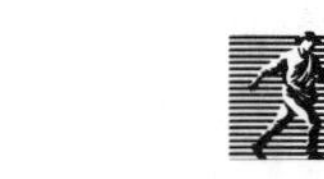

Prentice Hall
Upper Saddle River, NJ 07458

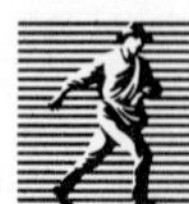

© 1999 by Prentice-Hall, Inc.
Simon & Schuster/A Viacom Company
Upper Saddle River, NJ 07458

10 9 8 7 6 5 4 3 2 1

ISBN 0-8359-5117-0
Printed in the United States of America

Contents

Introduction

From Nursing Assistant to Clinical Care Associate plunges into the exciting world of health care, especially that of the cross-trained, multiskilled unlicensed caregiver. Welcome! In addition to your textbook, you will find that this workbook has been designed as an aid for your success. With success as its focus, the workbook has been developed to interest you, to help you evaluate, and to involve you, the student, in the learning process.

This workbook is dependent upon and coordinated with the textbook, *From Nursing Assistant to Clinical Care Associate*. The workbook will guide you through your study of the textbook material. If you read something that puzzles you in the text or the workbook, ask your instructor to explain. Do not be afraid to ask questions. You should answer the workbook questions *after* you have read the chapter in the textbook. All the answers for the workbook questions are found within the text chapter.

The questions in this workbook were not written to stump, trick, or fool you. They were written to help you learn and review. Completing these workbook activities will fix the procedures and essential ideas firmly in your mind. Use these activities to become an active participant in the learning experiences.

A variety of exercises from crossword puzzles to multiple choice questions have been included, in an effort to meet your individual learning needs and to provide an effective learning experience that is compatible with your learning style. The knowledge and skill you gain will help you as you encounter a variety of experiences in your job.

Some tips for success as you study the text and use the workbook:

1. Take notes in an organized manner. Review your notes on a daily basis.
2. As you study, discover the various relationships, facts, definitions, rules, procedures, and skills that are presented.
3. Make an effort to avoid the trap of being bogged down with details. If you do not understand a concept, circle it, and come back to it later.

4. Try to work in small study groups to practice spelling, defining glossary terms, and covering the learning objectives at the beginning of the text chapter.
5. Be sure to keep up with the reading. If you get behind in the reading, you will have a difficult time during the instructor's lecture or demonstration.
6. You may wish to tape record specific terms or concepts that require extra attention. These tapes can then be played as you travel to and from school or run errands.

We hope you find these workbook activities to be useful and important tools. Enjoy!

C h a p t e r 1

The Health Care Environment

Chapter Review

Multiple Choice

1. Providing opportunities for health maintenance and health education programs is an example of __________ care.
   a. primary
   b. secondary
   c. tertiary
   d. quarternary

2. The primary consumers or customers of hospitals are
   a. visitors.
   b. patients.
   c. doctors.
   d. vendors.

3. Health measures aimed at treating illness to avoid hospitalization are
   a. primary.
   b. secondary.
   c. tertiary.
   d. quarternary.

4. Employees of a hospital can include all except
   a. nurses.
   b. plumbers.
   c. electricians.
   d. morticians.

5. Payment for hospital care is funded by all of the following sources except
   a. Medicare
   b. private insurance
   c. doctors
   d. private pay

6. DRG's targeted all except
   a. length of hospital stay.
   b. complications of surgery.
   c. unnecessary diagnostic procedures.
   d. cost of treatments per diagnosis.

7. Critical Pathways provide information about
   a. treatment costs.
   b. disease symptoms.
   c. outcome predictability.
   d. prescribed medications.

8. An on-site JCAHO visit will require review of all *but*
   a. management of care environment.
   b. documentation of patient assessment.
   c. data of patient education.
   d. report of financial standing.

9. Which of the following regulatory agencies ensures compliance with work safety and health codes?
   a. NRC
   b. OSHA
   c. JCAHO
   d. LSO

10. Performance improvement standards are instituted to
    a. ensure job efficiency.
    b. ensure OSHA regulations.
    c. measure care delivery.
    d. provide "ready to work" time.

11. The nursing model in which an RN delivers care to the patient during entire hospital stay is
    a. team.
    b. primary.
    c. holistic.
    d. multiskilled.

12. Which factor did NOT influence the reengineering of hospital care delivery?
    a. improve patient satisfaction
    b. maximize staff efficiency
    c. capture "ready to work time"
    d. increase number of providers

Vocabulary Activity

The following word search puzzle contains terms that are found in this chapter. Use the word list below to locate the hidden words in the grid.

```
U F I B L Q B X N K M S I P A H O U Q Z M B W B G
J I E C F F F H C N B U E U G E L U U B R C B M T
W C F A Y O X W R N S Q N L O A N E H P X R X Q M
T E A M N U R S I N G M O D E L N T I P D G D O X
R W W H G M K P B V J Y U C M T A R O I T A Q P T
G B H T O M A D R S I N O N V H M O S K M Q J M Q
R F A E Y A D S Q O S Y N U M C E G A E P T G D P
H G I V A P C G F J F U F O N A D H J Q R L L R L
T N J S K W F C A P Q I V E I R I F J P I H B V A
D J F B N O N P R O F I T P T E C N X B M B D G E
M N U R S E E X T E N D E R S S A P J O A O S F Q
E U Z I R B T A A L D E Y F J Q L O G A R J Z P R
P R I M A R Y N U R S I N G M O D E L Q Y J G O E
O S H A U W Q Q C D B I T E R T I A R Y C A R E Q
B I U U N O E C R I T I C A L P A T H W A Y R Q Q
R N Y K B P L Y O O R M A J T V G B P M R M K T P
X G E Q D M X Z S W L U F A Z I N C O H E P L K D
G P B R P L V S P Q G G D K J O O O L V F T C S P
D R G S W D Q E F A D R E V I Y S N W G O M G Y Q
K O C W Y K I E K S T E E J P D I S T L G Y A I Q
O C A L R V P Q U A L I T Y A S S U R A N C E P G
S E C O N D A R Y C A R E C P B S M K J A X I F G
U S G U T T F C W C B I R N K Z Y E O D A H J Y D
F S A A S A F Q X Q N E X U T V M R A F W S K D V
S T B L H D Z Z M A N W N T Z S M S U N C O D M T
```

1. consumers
2. critical pathway
3. DRGs
4. for-profit
5. health care
6. HMO
7. JCAHO
8. HCAHO Accreditation
9. medical diagnosis
10. nonprofit
11. NRC
12. nurse extenders
13. nursing processes
14. OSHA
15. patients
16. primary care
17. primary nursing model
18. quality assurance
19. secondary care
20. team nursing model
21. tertiary care

Developing Vocabulary

Writing Practice

Beside each word below, write a complete sentence using the word. For each sentence, check for accuracy of content, spelling, and punctuation.

1. patients ____

   ____

   ____

2. tertiary care ____

   ____

   ____

3. team nursing model ____

   ____

   ____

4. nonprofit ____

   ____

   ____

5. DRGs ____

   ____

6. primary nursing model ______________________________________

   ____

   ____

7. JCAHO Accreditation _______________________________________

   ____

   ____

8. consumers____

   ____

   ____

True or False

If the definition on the right corresponds to the word on the left, then check True; if the word and definition do not correspond, check False.

TRUE	FALSE	WORD
____	____	1. **Nonprofit:** organizations that provide services without capital
____	____	2. **Consumers:** customers of a particular business
____	____	3. **Quality assurance:** level of health care in which interventions are aimed at preventing illness and promoting wellness
____	____	4. **Medical diagnosis:** contracts with a medical group to care for its members, where doctors are rewarded for memer wellness
____	____	5. **Tertiary care:** level of health care in which interventions are implemented as a hospital admission

Spell Correctly

In each of the sets of words below, one word is spelled correctly. Circle the correctly spelled word.

1.   a. extunders   c. extinders
     b. extenders   d. extanders

2.   a. tertairy   c. tertiary
     b. tertiray   d. tertiury

3.   a. assurence   c. assurance
     b. assuronce   d. assuranue

4.   a. daignostic   c. diacnostic
     b. diagnostic   d. diagnestic

5.   a. reguletory   c. regulatory
     b. regilatory   d. regulatary

Practice Scenario(s)

After reading this chapter in the text, read the following scenario(s) and answer the questions following each of them.

Situation 1

Imagine that you work on a surgical floor in a hospital. Some post-operative (after surgery) patients who have had hysterectomies (removal of the uterus, or womb) are beginning to develop infections of the surgical incision. This is certainly not a desirable situation.

1. What do you think your surgical patient care unit should do?

____

____

____

2. What should the surgical patient care unit measure?

____

____

____

3. What data or information should be collected?

____

____

____

4. What information is needed to investigate and then solve this problem?

____

____

____

5. Suppose that the data for the above items have been collected for six months and the data must now be assessed. How would you assess the data?

____

____

____

6. How should the data be compared?

____

____

____

Care Delivery Alternatives

Chapter Review

Multiple Choice

1. Nursing homes, rehabilitation centers, and convalescent homes are considered __________ care facilities.
   - a. acute
   - b. long-term
   - c. primary
   - d. ambulatory

2. The consumers of long-term care are called
   - a. clients.
   - b. residents.
   - c. patients.
   - d. customers.

3. OBRA is a law that regulates
   - a. long-term care.
   - b. geriatric physicians.
   - c. community MH/MR.
   - d. medicare funding.

4. When was it mandated that nursing assistants in long-term care have certification?
   - a. 1979
   - b. 1997
   - c. 1987
   - d. 1990

5. The primary areas of OBRA legislation include all except
   - a. resident rights.
   - b. nurse aide registration.
   - c. resident assessment.
   - d. occupational safety.

6. All must be provided to long-term care residents under the Quality of Life provision of OBRA except
   - a. recreation.
   - b. socialization.
   - c. vision testing.
   - d. comforts of home.

7. Which of the following is the primary payment source for long-term care?
   a. HMO
   b. life insurance
   c. Medicare
   d. welfare

8. Of the following, which is NOT included in the resident assessment profile or MDS?
   a. cognitive loss
   b. rehab potential
   c. behavior symptoms
   d. demographic data

9. Community mental health and mental retardation services can be provided in
   a. long-term facilities.
   b. convalescent centers.
   c. vocational workshops.
   d. nursing homes.

10. Ambulatory care services are not offered in
    a. private physicians' offices.
    b. physician group practices.
    c. hospital-affiliated practices.
    d. home care agencies.

11. The Mental Health Law of 1979 influenced all except
    a. treatment methodology.
    b. rise in inpatient beds.
    c. integration in the community.
    d. release of patients from institutions.

12. In an ambulatory care setting, the multi-skilled CCA might perform which task?
    a. neurologic assessment
    b. history and physical
    c. breast exam
    d. electrocardiogram

13. Home care aides perform which of the following?
    a. coordinating services
    b. supervising paraprofessionals
    c. establishing plan of care
    d. assisting with ADL

14. Home care services may not be initiated for clients who are
    a. terminal.
    b. post hospital.
    c. rehabilitative.
    d. driving.

Vocabulary Activity

The following crossword puzzle contains terms that are found in this chapter. Use the clues below to complete the puzzle.

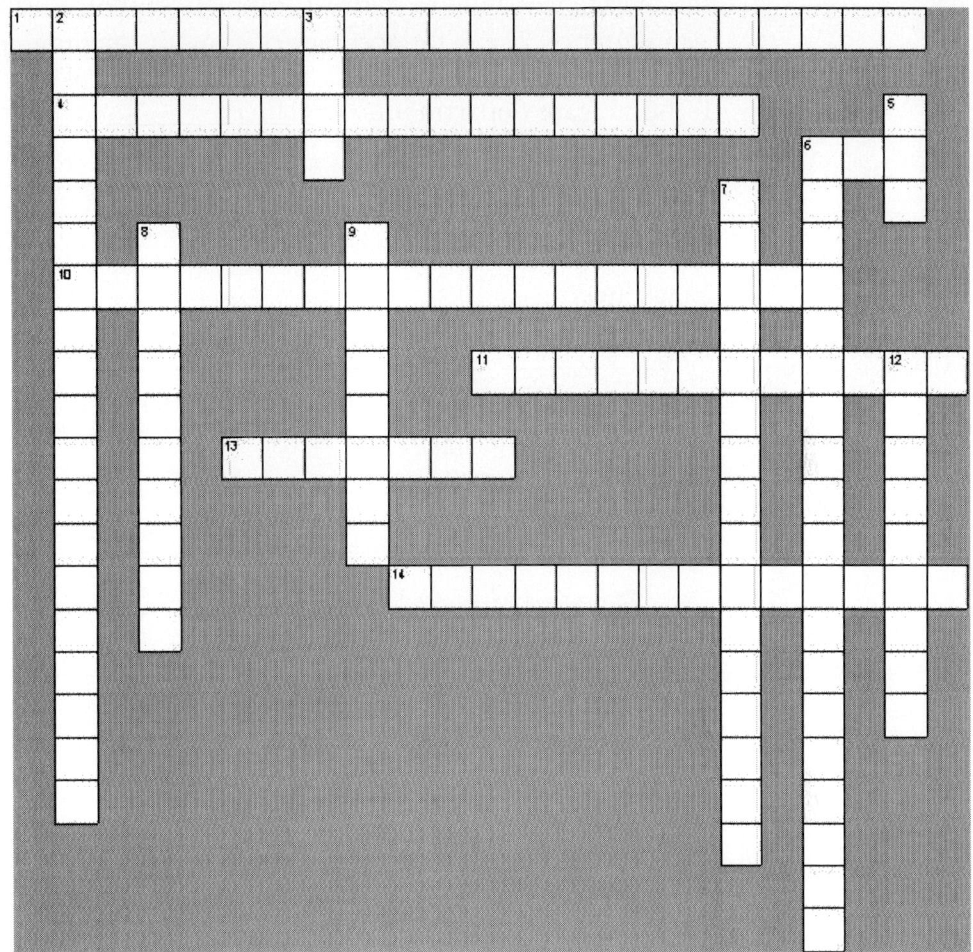

ACROSS

1. health care an individual receives in the community by "walking in"
4. RN with a master's degree in a specialty field of nursing
6. as needed/as necessary
10. department in hospitals that provides discharge planning to reduce poor transition
11. care of persons treated in nursing homes who will remain in the facility for a long period of time
13. outpatient, home care, or day clinic consumers of health-care services
14. standardized assessment that OBRA implemented to assure consistent resident evaluation nationally

DOWN

2. law that stimulated the closure of state mental hospitals and fostered outpatient care
3. law that regulates the business practices and care delivery of the long-term care industry
5. community-run organization that delivers health-care services to all segments of the health care continuum
6. licensed to perform physical examinations and to work with the doctor to treat patients
7. fee for service agreement
8. ability to walk
9. state of optimal health
12. title given to consumers of long-term care facilities

Developing Vocabulary

Writing Practice

Beside each word below, write a complete sentence using the word. For each sentence, check for accuracy of content, spelling, and punctuation.

1. home-care departments ______________________________________

   ____

   ____

2. wellness____

   ____

   ____

3. contractual basis ____

   ____

   ____

4. nurse practitioner ____

   ____

   ____

5. prn____

   ____

   ____

6. Mental Health Law of 1979 ____

   ____

   ____

7. OBRA ____

   ____

   ____

8. Minimum Data Set ____

   ____

   ____

True or False

If the definition on the right corresponds to the word on the left, then check True, if the word and definition do not correspond, check False.

TRUE   FALSE   WORD

____   ____   1. **VNA:** health care that an individual receives in the community by "walking in"

____   ____   2. **Clients:** law that regulates the business practices and care delivery of the long-term care industry

____   ____   3. **Miminum data set:** standardized assessment that OBRA implemented to assure consistent resident evaluation nationally

____   ____   4. **Physician's assistant:** outpatient, home care, or day clinic consumers of health-care services

____   ____   5. **Ambulatory:** ability to walk

Spell Correctly

In each of the sets of words below, one word is spelled correctly. Circle the correctly spelled word.

1.   a. contractuel   c. contractaul
       b. contractual   d. contrectual

2.   a. practationer   c. practetioner
       b. practitioner   d. practitooner

3.   a. association   c. associasion
       b. assocnation   d. assocaition

4.   a. omnibos   c. omnibus
       b. onmibus   d. omnibas

5.   a. reconcileation   c. reconciloation
       b. reconcilaition   d. reconciliation

Practice Scenario(s)

After reading this chapter in the text, read the following scenario(s) and answer the questions following each of them.

Situation 1

Your knowledge and understanding of the various types of care delivery alternatives, the way they function, and the regulatory agencies that govern them will form the basis for your interactions with staff and clients. Awareness of and adherence to specific state and facility- or agency-based procedures regarding client or patient care are your personal responsibility.

1. What motivated the legal enforcement of OBRA in the United States long-term care industry?

   ____

   ____

   ____

2. Why would you want to see the enforcement of OBRA for yourself or person that you love?

   ____

   ____

   ____

3. How would you explain the purpose of regulations, standards of care, and laws in the health-care industry?

   ____

   ____

   ____

4. Why do you think it is necessary for you to understand this information in your role as a clinical care associate?

   ____

   ____

   ____

5. Since you are not paid directly by the consumer or the insurance companies, why should you know about who pays and what the costs of heath care are?

   ____

   ____

   ____

6. Why do you think that patients, clients, and residents are called *customers* or *consumers?*

   ____

   ____

   ____

Emerging Health Care Roles

Chapter Review

Multiple Choice

1. All of the following terms are used to describe the expanded role of unlicensed care providers except
   a. multiskilled worker.
   b. registered technician.
   c. service worker.
   d. nursing associate.

2. Unlicensed care providers work under the supervision of
   a. physician assistants.
   b. nurse practitioners.
   c. licensed care providers.
   d. licensed psychologist.

3. Basic nursing assisting skills include all of the following except
   a. bathing.
   b. feeding.
   c. phlebotomy.
   d. ambulating.

4. In addition to assisting with ADL's, the home health aide may also perform which of the following tasks?
   a. light housekeeping
   b. gardening
   c. administering medications
   d. physical assessment

5. If you were interested in working as a resident counselor for an MH community agency, you should possess knowledge of
   a. mental illness.
   b. basic teaching skills.
   c. basic counseling.
   d. all of the above.

6. Which of the following health care providers must possess a license?
    a. M.D.
    b. C.N.A.
    c. C.C.A.
    d. U.A.P.

7. All of the following *licensed* team members would be on staff of an oncology unit except
    a. oncology clinical nurse specialist
    b. hematologist
    c. R.N.
    d. C.C.A.

8. The part of the computer that stores files within the computer is the
    a. hard drive.
    b. diskette.
    c. read-only memory.
    d. RAM

9. The handheld device that rolls on a hard surface and enables control of the computer is the
    a. hard drive.
    b. RAM.
    c. monitor.
    d. mouse.

10. Which of the following practitioners is a professional nurse?
    a. C.C.A.
    b. L.V.N.
    c. L.P.N.
    d. R.N.

Vocabulary Activity

The following crossword puzzle contains terms that are found in this chapter. Use the clues below to complete the puzzle.

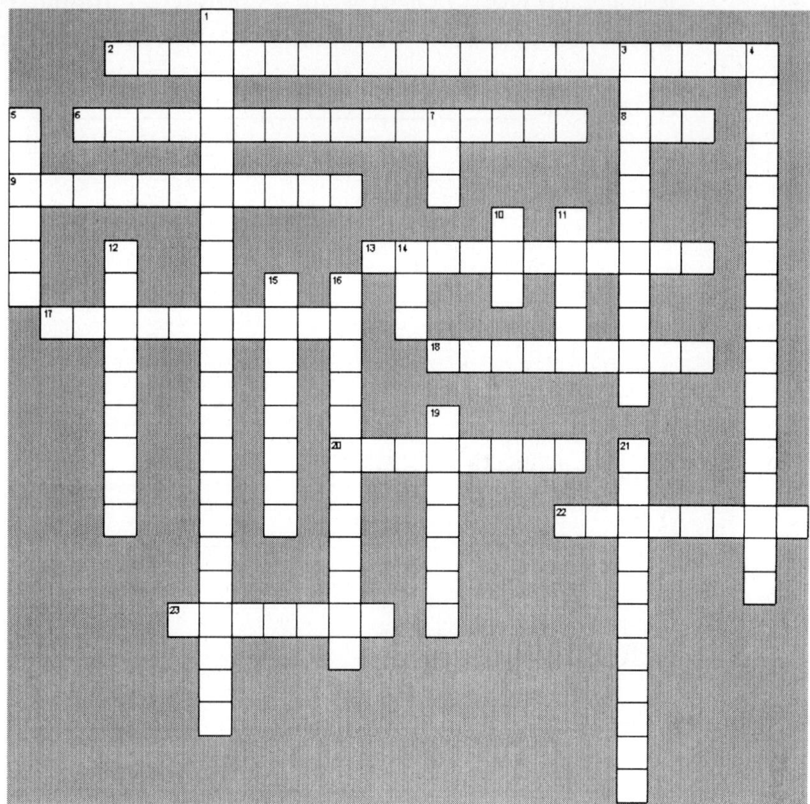

ACROSS

2. multiskilled worker who performs tasks of the nursing assistant and other extended skills
6. unlicensed assistant providing transport, housekeeping, and related duties
8. random access memory; temporary workspace memory
9. specialist who deals with skeletal diseases
13. physician who specializes in neurologic disorders
17. the port on the computer where CD's are inserted to run software
18. entering information into a designated software program
20. care of the patient with cancer
22. board linked to a computer on which typing is completed
23. professional document awarded following successful achievement of passing the state board exam

DOWN

1. individual who did not attend a prescribed academic/clinical program; assistive personnel
3. document, not a license, issued by an association to individuals who passed the association exam
4. a record of the electrical activity of the heart
5. turn on computer
7. computer's brain; central processing unit
10. read only memory; the permanent data saved as special programs that permit a computer to operate
11. hand-held device linked to a computer that rolls on a hard surface and controls computer functions by clicks
12. device that stores files within a computer
14. a record of the electrical activity of the heart
15. a three- and one-half-inch wafer cartridge that permits portable data storage
16. doctor who specializes in blood cell diseases
19. visual screen that displays the work completed on a computer
21. physician who specializes in physical rehab medicine

Developing Vocabulary

Writing Practice

Beside each word below, write a complete sentence using the word. For each sentence, check for accuracy of content, spelling, and punctuation.

1. boot up

2. CPU

3. neurologist

4. ROM

5. CD-ROM drive

6. data entry

7. keyboard

8. monitor

True or False

If the definition on the right corresponds to the word on the left, then check True, if the word and definition do not correspond, check False.

TRUE	FALSE	WORD
____	____	1. **Clinical care associate:** multiskilled worker who performs tasks of the nursing assistant and other extended skills.
____	____	2. **Certificate:** entering information into a designated software program
____	____	3. **Service associate:** unlicensed assistant providing transport, housekeeping, and related duties
____	____	4. **RAM:** document but not a license issued by an association to individuals who passed the association exam
____	____	5. **Hematologist:** doctor who specializes in blood cell diseases

Spell Correctly

In each of the sets of words below, one word is spelled correctly. Circle the correctly spelled word.

1.   a. deskette   c. diskitte
      b. diskette   d. diskotte

2.   a. physaitrist   c. phytiatrist
      b. physitarist   d. physiatrist

3.   a. orthopedizt   c. orthopedest
      b. orthopedast   d. orthopedist

4.   a. onoology   c. oncelogy
      b. oncology   d. oncilogy

5.   a. electrocardigoram   c. electrucardiogram
      b. electrocardiogram   d. eluctrocardiogram

Practice Scenario(s)

After reading this chapter in the text, read the following scenario(s) and answer the questions following each of them.

Situation 1

What are some reasons for the development of multiskill workers?

____

____

____

____

Situation 2

Which holds more weight, a license or a certificate?

____

____

____

____

Situation 3

Can a health-care provider hold a license and a certificate at the same time?

____

____

____

____

Situation 4

What data might a clinical care associate need to enter into a computer?

____

____

____

____

C h a p t e r   4

Health Care Employment

Chapter Review

Multiple Choice

1. A typewritten document that summarizes your work and educational background is a
   a. job description.
   b. transcript.
   c. cover letter.
   d. resume.

2. Which of the following information does not need to be included in your resume?
   a. age
   b. education
   c. experience
   d. address

3. Which of the following would NOT be an appropriate question to ask during a job interview?
   a. What shifts are available?
   b. What are the medical benefits?
   c. How long is the orientation?
   d. How much do you pay?

4. Which of the following is NOT a good source of job leads?
   a. clinical rotation site
   b. newspaper classifieds
   c. job posting in personnel
   d. relative employed in a company

5. A cover letter is a
   a. business letter accompanying a resume.
   b. personal note to thank the interviewer.
   c. narrative summary of your experience.
   d. required document with an application.

6. Which of the following skills is NOT essential for the CCA to possess?
   a. interpersonal
   b. critical thinking
   c. technical
   d. collegiate

7. Which of the following is true about delegation of tasks by the nurse to the clinical care associate?
   a. CCA can decline delegated tasks.
   b. Nurse assesses CCA's attitude.
   c. Delegation depends on patient's needs.
   d. Patient determines the delegation.

8. Federal law mandates that nursing assistants must be certified for which type of facility?
   a. community MH/MR
   b. long-term care
   c. home care
   d. ambulatory services

9. In which care setting does the assistant work with the nurse supervising from an off-site location?
   a. home
   b. hospital
   c. nursing home
   d. rehabilitation facility

10. After an interview, you should always
    a. shake hands to thank the interviewer.
    b. call the next day for an answer.
    c. send your resume to the interviewer.
    d. mail a brief cover letter.

11. An unlicensed care provider trained as a nursing assistant and performing expanded tasks is a
    a. practical nurse.
    b. patient care technician.
    c. respiratory assistant.
    d. physical therapy aide.

12. All of the following job titles are job leads for the CCA in community mental health except
    a. resident counselor.
    b. mental health counselor.
    c. resident advisor.
    d. behavior specialist.

13. When seeking a job in health care as an unlicensed assistant, you should expect to
    a. prepare a resume.
    b. forgo an application.
    c. interview the nurse.
    d. provide an action video.

14. If you are employed by a hospital as a clinical care associate, your immediate supervisor will be a
    a. practical nurse.
    b. medical social worker.
    c. registered nurse.
    d. practicing physician.

Vocabulary Activity

The following word search puzzle contains terms that are found in this chapter. Use the word list below to locate the hidden words in the grid.

```
E  J  F  U  X  B  V  G  L  W  W  Z  C  I  U  A  W  N  A  W
F  Z  N  W  S  D  N  W  X  W  J  P  F  U  F  J  G  I  Q  F
Y  L  A  I  P  F  B  E  C  H  G  D  D  A  O  L  E  G  D  K
V  T  H  A  J  O  B  B  R  H  E  K  A  D  F  M  S  T  K  G
D  C  Q  F  L  O  S  H  D  C  F  P  O  F  Z  Q  W  F  N  T
K  H  L  G  W  S  E  T  T  L  A  C  E  K  R  B  Z  Y  C  L
R  W  M  A  R  K  E  T  I  I  R  B  I  V  V  Z  B  K  F  X
U  T  Y  V  S  G  M  B  S  N  F  I  U  G  T  I  H  U  C  J
N  W  H  P  P  S  W  T  R  I  G  J  M  R  L  Z  C  L  A  Q
D  E  X  P  E  R  I  E  N  C  E  S  X  J  K  P  Y  F  P  D
Q  L  L  T  I  B  Z  F  H  A  X  F  I  R  I  Q  N  D  I  Z
E  M  P  L  O  Y  A  B  I  L  I  T  Y  F  O  R  L  F  B  K
Z  C  N  Y  O  I  X  E  N  E  T  W  O  R  K  I  N  G  W  K
Y  R  E  H  E  M  S  R  G  U  D  U  K  M  Y  U  U  U  J  U
K  G  Y  U  F  L  Q  U  R  R  E  S  U  M  E  D  J  O  A  P
K  P  L  W  Z  N  M  E  R  G  S  R  Y  P  X  J  S  K  A  J
V  P  W  Z  G  K  Z  Z  Q  K  M  J  D  S  R  V  M  K  O  S
K  K  X  I  K  Y  H  G  G  I  D  C  K  Q  Z  O  U  Z  H  B
C  D  N  Y  W  S  K  O  E  O  Q  Y  E  R  E  Q  X  G  D  Q
W  I  A  F  E  O  O  K  E  I  I  N  J  K  F  N  U  H  G  N
```

1. classifieds	6. market
2. clinical	7. networking
3. employability	8. postings
4. experiences	9. resume
5. job	

Developing Vocabulary

Writing Practice

Beside each word below, write a complete sentence using the word. For each sentence, check for accuracy of content, spelling, and punctuation.

1. employability _______________________________

    ____

    ____

2. networking _______________________________

    ____

    ____

3. resume _______________________________

    ____

    ____

4. postings _______________________________

    ____

    ____

5. clinical experiences

    ____

    ____

6. job _______________________________

    ____

    ____

7. market _______________________________

    ____

    ____

8. classifieds _______________________________

    ____

    ____

True or False

If the definition on the right corresponds to the word on the left, then check True, if the word and definition do not correspond, check False.

TRUE   FALSE   WORD

____   ____   1. **Networking:** section of the newspaper listing available and current jobs

____   ____   2. **Clinical experiences:** practice without pay in which certain skills are repeatedly performed

____   ____   3. **Market:** technique in which you sell your talents and abilities to gain employment

____   ____   4. **Resume:** brochure that lists your talents and abilities for an employer

____   ____   5. **Job postings:** listing of jobs available within the health-care system visibly displayed in the personnel department

Spell Correctly

In each of the sets of words below, one word is spelled correctly. Circle the correctly spelled word.

1.   a. clenical experience   c. clinucal experience
      b. clinical experience   d. clinipal experience

2.   a. murket   c. market
      b. marmet   d. merket

3.   a. netwerking   c. notworking
      b. nteworking   d. networking

4.   a. rasume   c. resume
      b. resime   d. risume

5.   a. clissifieds   c. classifeids
      b. classifieds   d. clessifieds

Practice Scenario(s)

After reading this chapter in the text, read the following scenario(s) and answer the questions following each of them.

Situation 1

Imagine that you are going on a job interview for a home health aide (HHA) position. You have just completed a CNA course but have never had a job in health care.

1. How will you describe your ability to fulfill the requirements of the role?

____

____

____

Situation 2

Review Table 4-1 *Interview Between Inez and Mrs. Potts* in your text.

1. How did Inez know about the company's reputation?

____

____

____

2. Why didn't Inez state that she might go back to school in five years for a psychology degree?

____

____

____

3. Why didn't Inez mention her habit of sleeping through her alarm as one of her weaknesses?

____

____

____

Medical Terms and Abbreviations

Chapter Review

Multiple Choice

1. The foundation or major word component of a medical term is the
   a. suffix.
   b. word root.
   c. prefix.
   d. combining part.

2. A __________ is found at the end of a medical term.
   a. prefix
   b. suffix
   c. combining form
   d. word root

3. Itis means
   a. condition.
   b. tumor.
   c. inflammation.
   d. knowledge.

4. Gastro means
   a. stomach.   c. intestine.
   b. colon.   d. bladder.

5. Pathology is the study of
   a. disease.   c. cancer.
   b. conditions.   d. cells.

6. Polydipsia means
   a. without digestion.
   b. excessive thirst.
   c. difficult swallowing.
   d. overeating.

7. The term for fear of light is
   a. photophobia.
   b. olfactophobia.
   c. ophthalmophobia.
   d. phonophobia.

8. The term for lack of speech is
   a. dysphagia.
   b. bradypepsin.
   c. tachypnea.
   d. aphasia.

9. Medical shorthand for documentation or dictation of patient information is medical
   a. terminology.
   b. abbreviations.
   c. charting.
   d. records.

10. The medical abbreviation for an infection in the urinary system is
    a. URI.   c. UBI.
    b. UTI.   d. URT.

11. FUO means
    a. fever of unknown origin.
    b. fungus with unknown outcome.
    c. fulminating urinary output.
    d. from urinary obstruction.

12. If a patient is permitted to use the bathroom, the doctor's order would contain which abbreviation?
    a. BRP   c. BR
    b. HOB   d. BRO

13. The doctor's order reads: Tylenol 650 mg. P.O. q4h. P.R.N. headache. What does P.R.N. indicate in this order?
    a. per registered nurse
    b. permission required now
    c. whenever possible
    d. as needed

14. The abbreviation for stroke is
    a. CVA.   c. CMI.
    b. MI.   d. CMA.

15. Costochondritis refers to swelling of
    a. ileum and bones.
    b. ligaments and muscles.
    c. ribs and cartilage.
    d. tendons and joints.

Vocabulary Activity

The following word search puzzle contains terms that are found in this chapter. Use the word list below to locate the hidden words in the grid.

```
C A R D I O L O G Y C N G L E T R A X G
J O H K T C M G S H R N Y A U V A L R Q
M Z M E O G Y K E U E E J W U K R M V A
V B S B S L P W G F V P H G V D H D T U
J E D F I N O C T U R I A H P Q Y U G J
S J W A E N D O C A R D I T I S F J E A
B N P R E F I X S D G A S B I U K A A T
W H N B L L I N E P H R O P A T H Y N H
I A E H Y P E R G L Y C E M I A I D T H
B S U F F I X U T V S S C L E R O S I S
T M R R G W N R K G O Q O D H F T R G P
F C O A A H Z F E O K W L N Q I M W E M
I P P R S E F K Y M C P E X C I B T N Z
G G A S T R O S T O M Y C L L E R J X T
O Y T E R Y T H R O C Y T E H D O Q W X
H T H R O M B O S I S D O O S F P R L G
K F Y G T I L E O S T O M Y S K P R M P
T S G W O R D R O O T I Y K Y I D O A S
C D H E M I P L E G I A X H J F S I M Y
T M P N Y D Y X I W V N P A Q I Q I A X
```

1. antigen	12. ileostomy
2. cardiology	13. leukocytosis
3. colectomy	14. nephropathy
4. combining vowel	15. neuropathy
5. endocarditis	16. nocturia
6. erythrocyte	17. prefix
7. gastrostomy	18. sclerosis
8. gastrotomy	19. suffix
9. hemiplegia	20. thrombosis
10. hepatitis	21. word root
11. hyperglycemia	

Developing Vocabulary

Writing Practice

Beside each word below, write a complete sentence using the word. For each sentence, check for accuracy of content, spelling, and punctuation.

1. erythrocyte ____

   ____

   ____

2. suffix ____

   ____

   ____

3. nocturia ____

   ____

   ____

4. nephropathy ____

   ____

   ____

5. antigen ____

   ____

   ____

6. neuropathy ____

   ____

   ____

7. hepatitis ____

   ____

   ____

8. leukocytosis ____

   ____

   ____

True or False

If the definition on the right corresponds to the word on the left, then
check True, if the word and definition do not correspond, check False.

TRUE	FALSE	WORD
____	____	1. **Prefix:** a word that begins a word
____	____	2. **Combining vowel:** condition of hardening
____	____	3. **Gastrotomy:** the study of the heart
____	____	4. **Colectomy:** a vowel, usually O, that connects word parts
____	____	5. **Hyperglycemia:** above normal blood sugar

Spell Correctly

In each of the sets of words below, one word is spelled correctly. Circle
the correctly spelled word.

1.
   a. thrembosis
   b. thrombotis
   c. thrombosis
   d. thrumbosis

2.
   a. sclirosis
   b. sclerosas
   c. sclreosis
   d. sclerosis

3.
   a. ileostomy
   b. ileistomy
   c. ileostoly
   d. ileostumy

4.
   a. hemiplegea
   b. himiplegia
   c. hemiplegia
   d. hemiplegua

5.
   a. endocardetis
   b. endocarditis
   c. endocardisis
   d. endocarditus

Practice Scenario(s)

After reading this chapter in the text, read the following scenario(s) and answer the questions following each of them.

Situation 1

You attend a seminar to upgrade your skills. The topic is patient care for tracheostomy.

1. What is a tracheostomy?

    ____

    ____

    ____

2. What is the difference between tracheotomy and tracheostomy?

    ____

    ____

    ____

3. Why would a patient have a tracheostomy?

    ____

    ____

    ____

Situation 2

Today you are pulled to the urology floor. The first patient report you receive is about Mr. Harrison, who has suprapubic cystotomy. The next patient has chronic nephritis and is now on hemodialysis.

1. To what floor are you going?

    ____

    ____

    ____

2. What is suprapubic cystotomy?

____

____

____

3. What is nephritis?

____

____

____

4. What is hemodialysis?

____

____

____

Situation 3

Mr. Byrns, a longtime resident of your nursing home, was taken to the hospital for surgery of a malignant melanoma L shoulder. What is melanoma?

____

____

____

____

Situation 4

Mrs. McCartney is a 43 yo W ♀ adm $\bar{c}$ severe pain RLQ, N&V, r/o appendicitis. What does this mean to you?

____

____

____

____

Situation 5

Mrs. Sandeler has just returned $\bar{p}$ a L Lobectomy for carcinoma. What is a lobectomy?

1. What is a lobectomy?

____

____

____

2. What is carcinoma?

____

____

____

Situation 6

You received A.M. report from the nurse. Mr. Lennon a 75 yo ♂ adm last night $\bar{c}$ c/o severe dyspnea, + pedal edema, and bibasilar rales. Dx R/O CHF. He is on cont O_2 @ 2L/min. via nasal cannula. He requires pulse check at 9 A.M. Report results STAT to RN. He can be OOB ad lib $\bar{c}$ BRP. HOB ↑ 45° at all times. He has a history of COPD. What should you do for Mr. Lennon today?

____

____

____

____

Situation 7

The nurse informs you to check the nursing Kardex for an update on the pt.'s nursing orders and ADL status. These are your findings: NG tube to suction, NPO, $\bar{c}$ sips of H_2O, IV ® arm, BR. What does this mean to you?

____

____

____

____

Situation 8

Mr. Stark is adm with oliguria, hematuria, and dysuria. IVP reveals pyelonephritis. What does this mean?

____

____

____

____

Situation 9

You took a position $\bar{c}$ a MH/MR agency as a residential supervisor of three males in a half-way house. All the clients are in their 50's. One client has acromegaly, one has dyskinesia, and one is dysphasic.

1. What can you expect from each one?

____

____

____

2. Since acromegaly enlarges the extremities including the hands and feet, from what problems might this client suffer?

____

____

____

Situation 10

As a HHA, you are called by the nursing supervisor to cover four Medicare cases today. The nurse give you TO and tells you to √ the care plan in each home. The first client suffers from IDDM. She requires asst $\bar{c}$ transfer to shower. She tells you to avoid bumping her legs because she suffers from polyneuropathy. The second case is a L CVA $\bar{c}$ ® hemiplegia and aphasia. He is being seen by PT, ST, OT, RN, and HHA. The care plan in the home states the HHA is to assist with ROM. The third case is a client $\bar{c}$ a colostomy 2° colorectal CA.

The fourth client is being followed by home care after an acute anterolateral myocardial infarction with subsequent necrosis.

1. What is IDDM?

2. What are you expected to do regarding the client's need for assistance with transfer to shower?

3. From your understanding of medical terminology, what is polyneuropathy?

4. What does "L CVA $\bar{c}$ ® hemiplegia and aphasia" mean?

5. Regarding the second client mentioned in this scenario, who is following this client at home?

6. What does it mean that the HHA is to assist with ROM?

7. What does the following tell you? "The third case is a client c̄ a colostomy 2° colorectal CA."

8. What does anterolateral mean?

9. What does myocardial mean?

10. What is necrosis?

Chapter 6
The Body as a Whole

Chapter Review

Multiple Choice

1. The science that deals with the study of the functions of the human body is called
   a. anatomy.
   b. biology.
   c. pathology.
   d. physiology.

2. Which part of the cell acts as a boundary between the cell and the environment outside the cell?
   a. cytoplasm
   b. nucleus
   c. cell membrane
   d. cell wall

3. Genetic information is stored in a cellular molecule called
   a. organelle.
   b. RNA.
   c. mitosis.
   d. DNA.

4. The cytoplasm of the cell contains
   a. organelles.
   b. water.
   c. minerals.
   d. all of the above

5. Genes align themselves on structures called
   a. genetic bands.
   b. chromosomes.
   c. offspring.
   d. DNA.

6. The three main parts of a cell are
    a. cell membrane, nucleus, cytoplasm.
    b. cell membrane, genes, protoplasm.
    c. mitochondria, cell membrane, cytoplasm.
    d. cytoplasm, brain, cell wall.

7. Which type of cells continually replicate or reproduce themselves?
    a. red blood cells
    b. hepatocytes
    c. muscle cells
    d. nerve cells

8. Cells of similiar function unite to form
    a. tissues.
    b. organs.
    c. cytoplasm.
    d. systems.

9. What type of tissue is fibrous and acts to hold the structures of the body together?
    a. epithelial
    b. connective
    c. muscular
    d. nervous

10. Which of the following is both a system and an organ?
    a. blood
    b. skeleton
    c. skin
    d. liver

11. Which term refers to the back of the body or of a structure?
    a. cephalic
    b. caudal
    c. ventral
    d. dorsal

12. Imaginary lines that can be drawn horizontally and vertically to separate the abdomen into four parts are called
    a. cavities.   c. systems.
    b. planes.   d. quadrants.

13. The trachea, larynx, pharynx, and bronchi are organs of the
    ___________ system.
    a. digestive   c. endocrine
    b. reproductive   d. respiratory

14. Tissues are joined together to form
    a. systems.   c. organs.
    b. membranes.   d. cavities.

Identification Exercise

Label the figure below:

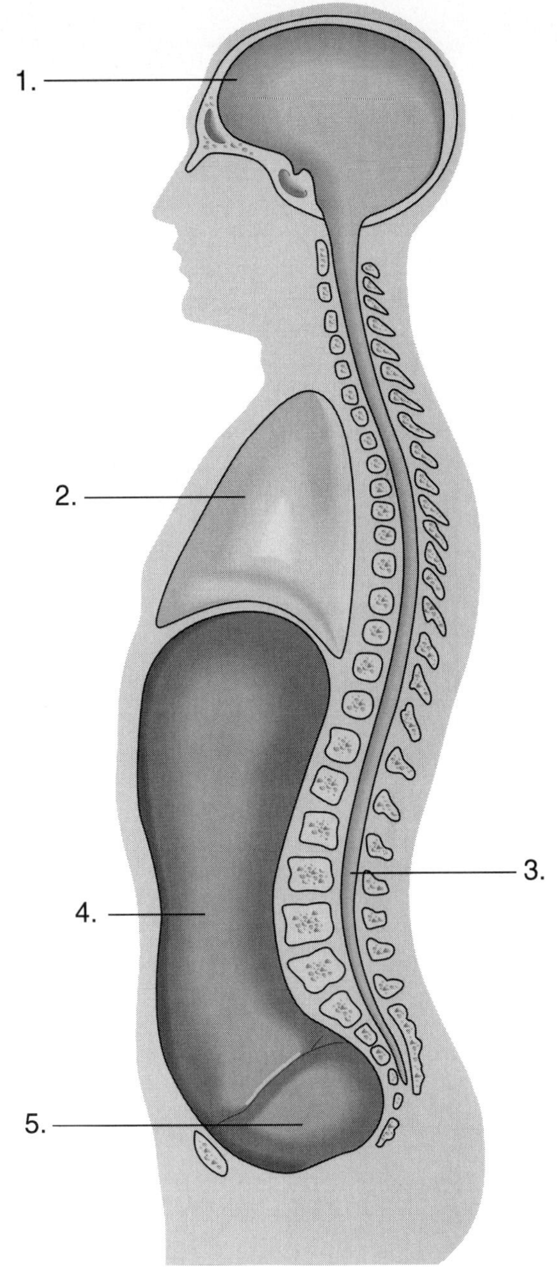

1. _______________________

2. _______________________

3. _______________________

4. _______________________

5. _______________________

Vocabulary Activity

The following crossword puzzle contains terms that are found in this chapter. Use the clues below to complete the puzzle.

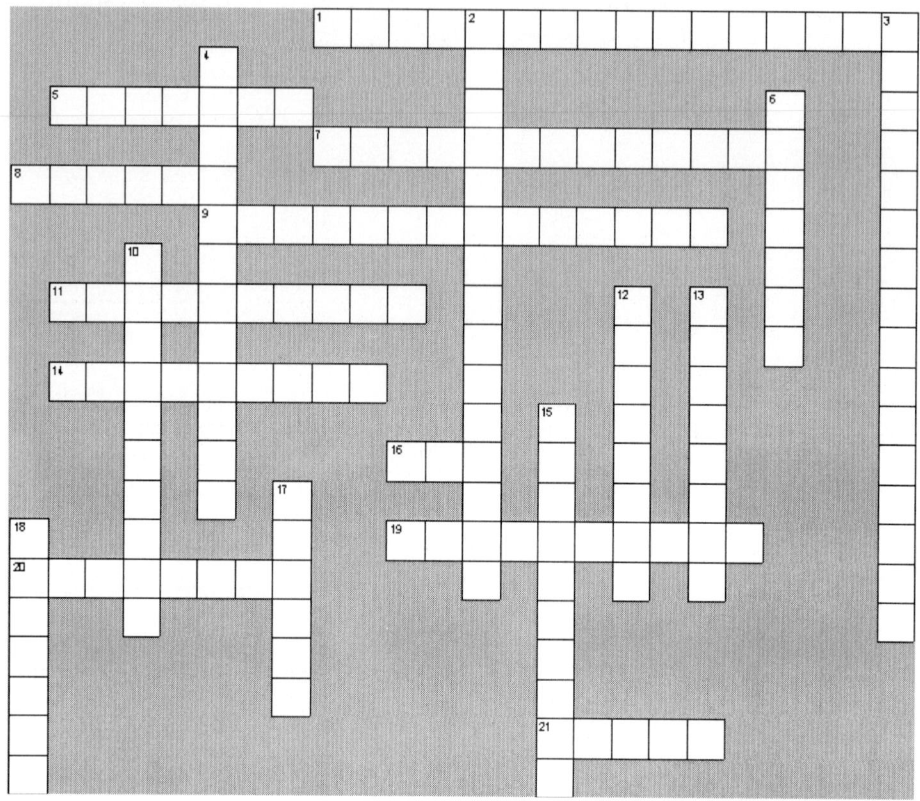

ACROSS

1. includes the fibrous tissue that holds the body together
5. the brain of the cell; directs all of the cellular activities
7. composed of nerve cells called neurons
8. pertaining to the middle or midline
9. composed of special cells designed to contract to produce movement
11. one of the bodies in the cell nucleus that carries genes
14. imaginary scoring of the abdomen into 4 circular areas
16. ladder of amino acids that form a genetic code
19. is made up of various organs that act together to produce specific functions of the body
20. ventral or front side of the body or structure
21. contain the heritage of each organism passed on to individuals by their ancestors

DOWN

2. glands that have no ducts; their secretions are absorbed directly into the blood
3. tissue designed to secrete and absorb substances
4. thin layer of cells that act as a boundary between the cell contents and the outside environment
6. belly side of an animal
10. structures that carry out digestive, respiratory, and circulatory functions
12. a life-form; a living being made of many structures that are dependent on one another
13. chemical messenger secreted by endocrine glands
15. study of the function of the organism
17. posterior or back side of the body
18. pertaining to the side; farthest from the midline

Developing Vocabulary

Writing Practice

Beside each word below, write a complete sentence using the word. For each sentence, check for accuracy of content, spelling, and punctuation.

1. cell ___________________________________

   ____

   ____

2. flagella _______________________________

   ____

   ____

3. genes _________________________________

   ____

   ____

4. genetic code _____________________________

   ____

   ____

5. inferior _______________________________

   ____

   ____

6. mitosis ________________________________

   ____

   ____

7. organelles ______________________________

   ____

   ____

8. system _________________________________

   ____

   ____

True or False

If the definition on the right corresponds to the word on the left, then check True, if the word and definition do not correspond, check False.

TRUE	FALSE	WORD
____	____	1. **Hormones:** chemical messenger secreted by endocrine glands.
____	____	2. **Epithelial tissue:** made up of various organs that act together to produce specific functions of the body
____	____	3. **Nervous tissue:** composed of nerve cells called neurons
____	____	4. **Anterior:** study of the function of the organism
____	____	5. **Endocrine glands:** glands that have no ducts; their secretions are absorbed directly into the blood

Spell Correctly

In each of the sets of words below, one word is spelled correctly. Circle the correctly spelled word.

1. a. medail   c. medual
    b. medial   d. mediel

2. a. laaeral   c. laterol
    b. lateral   d. leteral

3. a. anatomy   c. ananomy
    b. anatamy   d. anayomy

4. a. chremosome   c. coromosome
    b. chromosome   d. chromasome

5. a. organism   c. orgainsm
    b. orgaaism   d. orgnaism

Practice Scenario(s)

After reading this chapter in the text, read the following scenario(s) and answer the questions following each of them.

Situation 1

Your patient has right upper quadrant pain.

1. Exactly where is the patient's pain?

____

____

____

Situation 2

The physician's order reads for a posterior/lateral x-ray of the thorax.

1. What body part will be x-rayed?

____

____

____

Situation 3

The lateral bone of the forearm is fractured at the distal end of the bone.

1. Exactly where has this fracture occurred?

____

____

____

Situation 4

A patient is told that a mass was found in the pelvic cavity.

1. Describe where this mass is located.

____

____

____

Situation 5

You are instructed to swab a patient's wound for cytology studies.

1. What laboratory will receive this specimen?

____

____

____

The Skin

Chapter Review

Multiple Choice

1. The skin is referred to as the_____________ system.
   a. skeletal
   b. integumentary
   c. muscular
   d. dermal

2. Characteristics of the epidermis include all except
   a. contains melanin.
   b. is composed of cells that continually shed and reproduce.
   c. is the uppermost layer of the skin.
   d. contains blood vessels.

3. The chemical substance that produces skin pigment is
   a. melanocyte.
   b. membrane color.
   c. melanin.
   d. epidermal pigment.

4. What is needed to protect the skin from the harmful rays of the sun?
   a. melanin
   b. sunscreen
   c. ultraviolet light
   d. vitamin D

5. The dermis is composed of _____________ tissue.
   a. connective
   b. epidermal
   c. subcutaneous
   d. epithelial

6. The dermis contains all except
   a. blood vessels.
   b. nerves.
   c. sweat glands.
   d. melanin.

7. Which glands help to moisturize the skin?
   a. endocrine glands
   b. sweat glands
   c. oil glands
   d. arrectores pilorum

8. Which glands help to cool the human body?
   a. oil
   b. sweat
   c. salivary
   d. endocrine

9. Which of the following is not a function(s) of intact skin?
   a. control body temperature from evaporation of sweat
   b. alert the body to harmful or pleasurable sensations
   c. produces pigment
   d. provide opportunity for infection

10. A condition commonly referred to as pimples is
    a. psoriasis
    b. scabies
    c. acne
    d. pressure sores

11. First-degree burns involve injury to the
    a. dermis.
    b. epidermis.
    c. adipose tissue.
    d. subcutaneous tissue.

12. Hives are
    a. usually the result of an allergic reaction.
    b. are raised patches that are white in the center and raised at
       the edges.
    c. itchy.
    d. all of the above

13. A third-degree burn involves injury to all but
    a. the epidermis.
    b. dermis.
    c. adipose.
    d. bone.

14. What can cause skin breakdown?
    a. immobility because of the pressure of body weight on bony
       prominences
    b. "onion" skin
    c. wrinkles
    d. being overweight

Identification Exercise

Label the figure below:

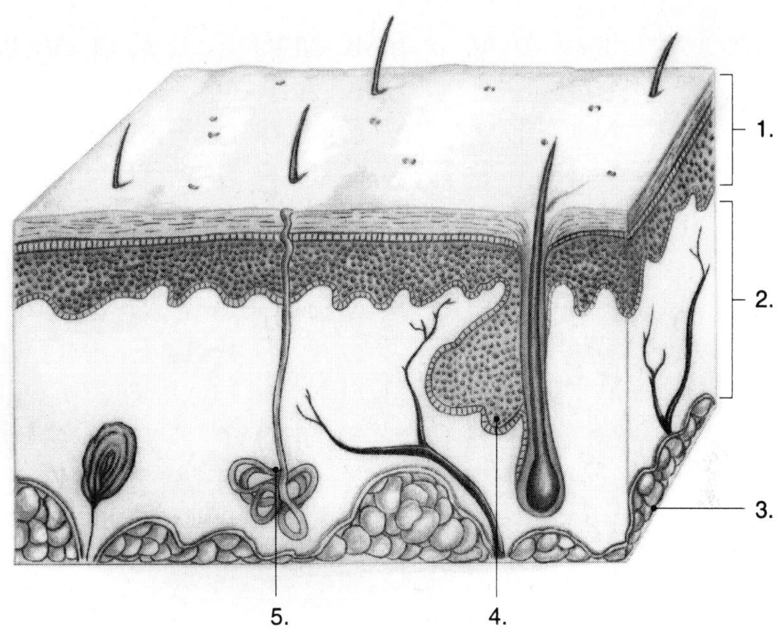

1.______________________________

2.______________________________

3.______________________________

4.______________________________

5.______________________________

Vocabulary Activity

The following word search puzzle contains terms that are found in this chapter. Use the word list below to locate the hidden words in the grid.

```
I V V V J R K M W E L G I V L R N I K G
C N E E Q M K Z F V Z N Y X T N O V O G
N C T Z I V D W G G F S V B Y A A S A T
H R T E S K Q A P E E B N C U F W R R G
W E Y H G Z N W W T B V V Y Q G P K R C
E P C M I U M A V N T W W E P A C N E H
E P I D E R M I S G E S D A R D S U C D
F I R S T - D E G R E E B U R N S Q T R
J T R V K D U - N U V X K O D K Y U O U
G C P H Q K Y M D T S U M G V Q D H R G
K V W S F Q X P I E A Z X B G V H H E X
U S E C O N D - D E G R E E B U R N S C
D U O D E R M I S Q C R Y R J D U T P D
C Y A N O S I S B H I V E S P Q R I I Z
U W S Y M E L A N I N M T E Y G A F L K
W Z I P V B K Q S Y P C S R B S W E O E
U P S A L I K F C I X P W E H U T Y R C
N Y B G R P B D M H S Y P Z O L R E U M
J Y A Q C Q C Q I P Y Q G L D C T N M I
Q F Z G D E C U B I T U S U L C E R S V
```

1. acne
2. arrectores pilorum
3. cyanosis
4. decubitus ulcers
5. dermis
6. duoderm
7. epidermis
8. first-degree burns
9. hives
10. integumentary system
11. melanin
12. psoriasis
13. second-degree burns
14. third-degree burns

Developing Vocabulary

Writing Practice

Beside each word below, write a complete sentence using the word. For each sentence, check for accuracy of content, spelling, and punctuation.

1. decubitus ulcers ______________________________________

____

____

2. second-degree burns ______________________________________

____

____

3. epidermis ______________________________________

____

____

4. psoriasis______________________________________

____

____

5. arrectores pilorum ______________________________________

____

____

6. hives ______________________________________

____

____

7. melanin______________________________________

____

____

8. integumentary system______________________________________

____

____

True or False

If the definition on the right corresponds to the word on the left, then check True, if the word and definition do not correspond, check False.

TRUE   FALSE   WORD

____   ____   1. **Second-degree burns:** noninfectious, chronic inflammatory skin disease

____   ____   2. **Cyanosis:** bluish coloration of the skin

____   ____   3. **Arrectores pilorum:** partial thickness involving dermal injury causing blisters

____   ____   4. **Epidermis:** superficial burns that involve injury to the epidermis only

____   ____   5. **Decubitus ulcers:** muscle fibers that help to keep the heat in the body

Spell Correctly

In each of the sets of words below, one word is spelled correctly. Circle the correctly spelled word.

1.   a. psoriasis   c. psuriasis
       b. psoraisis   d. psiriasis

2.   a. derris   c. dermis
       b. durmis   d. dremis

3.   a. cyaonsis   c. cynaosis
       b. cyenosis   d. cyanosis

4.   a. duodirm   c. duodrem
       b. duiderm   d. duoderm

5.   a. arractores pilorum   c. arrectores pilorum
       b. arrecteres pilorum   d. arrictores pilorum

Practice Scenario(s)

After reading this chapter in the text, read the following scenario(s) and answer the questions following each of them.

Situation 1

If you were to take residents in your LTC facility to a picnic on a hot summer day, you would need to consider another potential risk. The risk is not related to the UV rays of the sun, but the effects of heat.

1. What would you observe about the skin in relation to being outdoors on a summer day?

____

____

____

Situation 2

In your work, you should always notice the patient's skin color and any changes in it.

1. What would you do if you noticed that a patient's skin color was flushed, or if the skin tone changed to a gray or bluish color?

____

____

____

Situation 3

Consider the factors that lead to skin breakdown and pressure sores.

1. What actions can you take as a clinical care associate to prevent the development of decubitus ulcers?

____

____

____

Situation 4

Using your current knowledge of nutrition, consider the following.

1. What should you encourage patients to eat to heal damaged skin?

    ____

    ____

    ____

2. If you are unsure about nutritional factors and their effect on maintaining healthy skin, what member of the health care team can provide the answers?

    ____

    ____

    ____

Chapter 8

The Skeletal System

Chapter Review

Multiple Choice

1. Calcium is stored in all but the __________ bones.
   a. striated
   b. short
   c. irregular
   d. flat

2. An example of a long bone is the
   a. femur.
   b. hyoid.
   c. sternum.
   d. occiput.

3. The central shaft of a long bone is called the
   a. epiphysis.
   b. diaphysis.
   c. red marrow.
   d. cancellous tissue.

4. The part of the skeletal system that includes the arms, legs, hands, and feet is the __________ skeleton.
   a. axial.
   b. true.
   c. appendicular.
   d. false.

5. The bones of the neck are called the __________ vertebrae.
   a. lumbar.
   b. thoracic.
   c. sacral.
   d. cervical.

6. The normal curve of the lumbar section of the spine is
   described as
   a. kyphotic.   c. concave.
   b. convex.   d. lordotic.

7. The term used to describe an abnormal curve of the thorax is
   a. thoracosis.   c. lordosis.
   b. kyphosis.   d. scoliosis.

8. The long bone of the upper arm is the
   a. humerus.
   b. tibia.
   c. ulna.
   d. radius.

9. The bones of the wrists are collectively called the
   a. tarsals.
   b. calcanea.
   c. carpals.
   d. metacarpals.

10. Freely movable joints are found in all except
    a. hips.
    b. shoulders.
    c. ribs.
    d. carpals.

11. The articulation of two bones is called
    a. tendon.
    b. cartilage.
    c. a ligament
    d. joint.

12. The functions of the skeletal system include all but
    a. framework.
    b. protection.
    c. support.
    d. movement.

13. Where are blood cells produced?
    a. calcium-storing cells
    b. bone marrow
    c. diaphysis
    d. muscle tissue

14. Which of the following is the most common chronic condition
    of older Americans?
    a. osteoarthritis
    b. rheumatoid arthritis
    c. osteoporosis
    d. herniated intervertebral discs

Identification Exercise

Label the figure below:

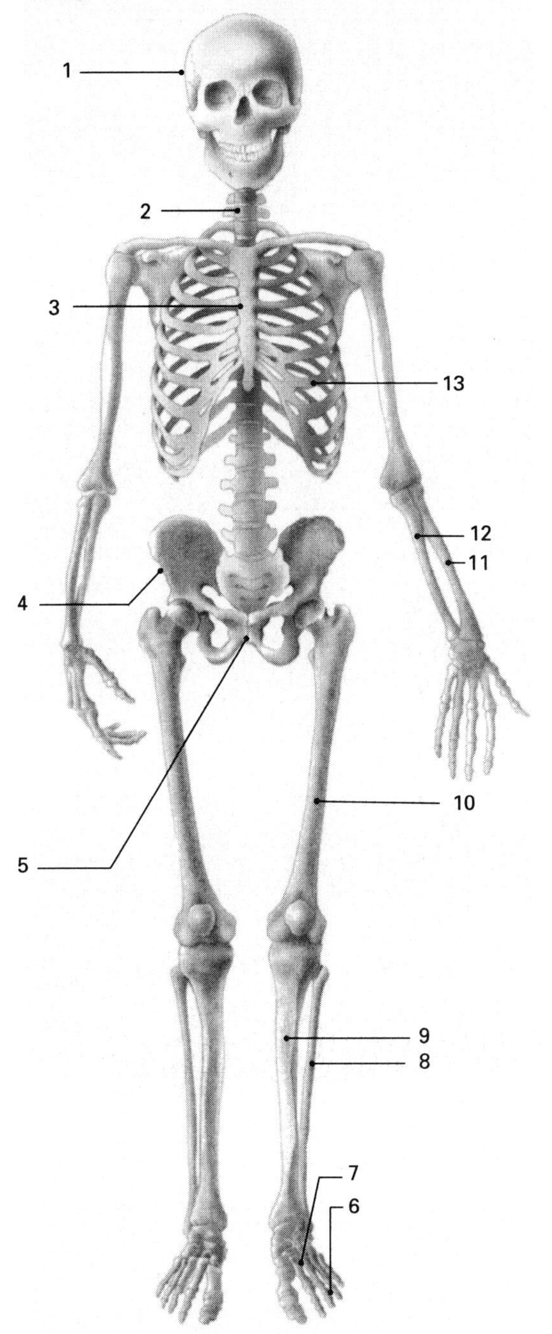

1. _______________________

2. _______________________

3. _______________________

4. _______________________

5. _______________________

6. _______________________

7. _______________________

8. _______________________

9. _______________________

10. _______________________

11. _______________________

12. _______________________

13. _______________________

Vocabulary Activity

The following crossword puzzle contains terms that are found in this chapter. Use the clues below to complete the puzzle.

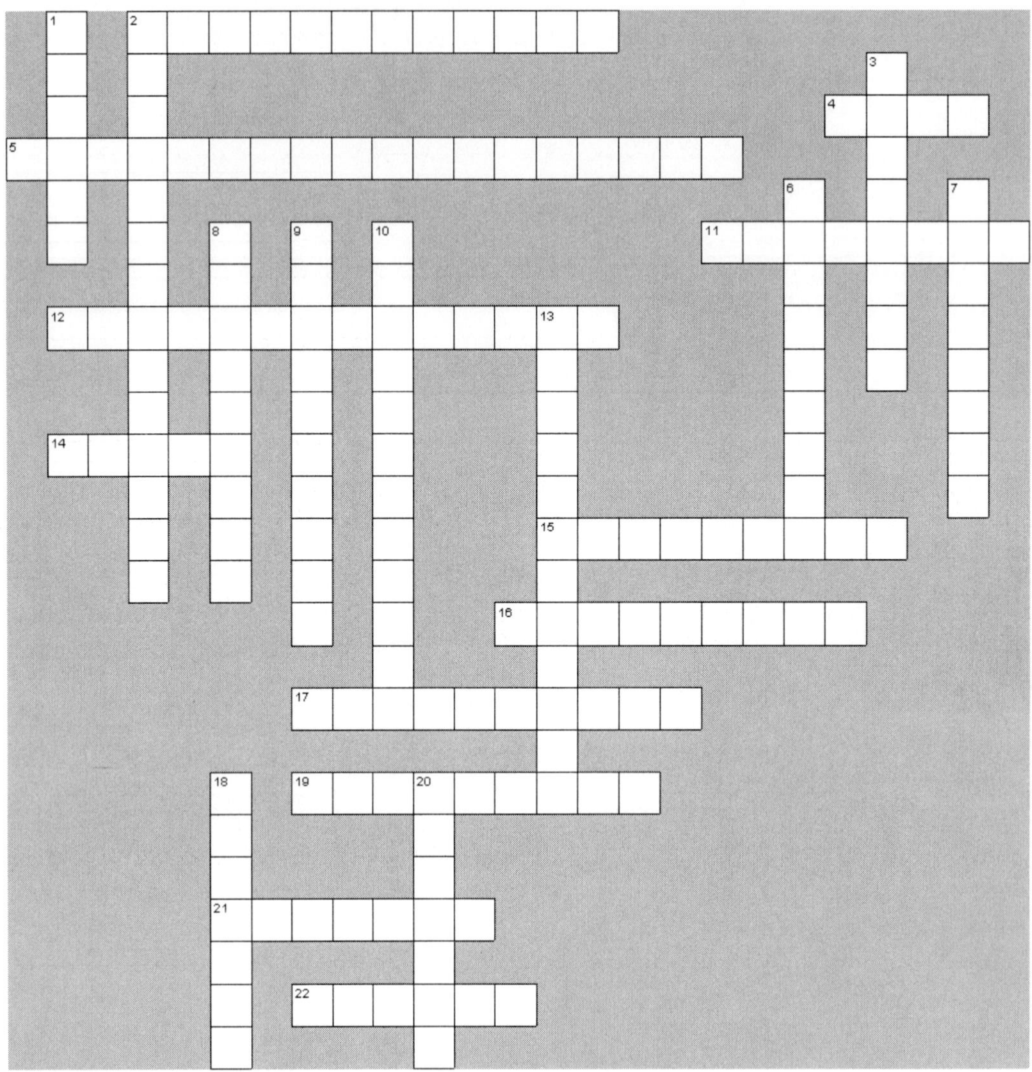

ACROSS

2. loss of bone calcium, causing brittle bones and spontaneous fractures
4. painful form of arthritis or joint inflammation caused by the deposit of uric acid around the joint
5. cushion between each vertebra of the spine that helps to absorb shock and prevent friction
11. abnormal curve of the thoratic vertebrae of the spine
12. between the spinal bones
14. subdivision of the skeletal system that includes the bones of the cranium, face, spinal column, and the chest
15. the central shaft of the long bones
16. sideway curvature of any section of the vertebral spine
17. bone tissue that is spongy and porous
19. broken bones
21. bone tissue that is dense and strong
22. spinal areas that curve outward

DOWN

1. the unions of two or more bones; also called articulation
2. inflammation of the joints occurring as a result of aging
3. exaggerated concave or anterior curve of the lumbar area of the spine
6. each end of the long bone
7. tough, fibrous band of connective tissue that connects one bone to another
8. tough connective tissue that covers the ends of the bones
9. arthritis-like
10. union of two or more bones
13. subdivision of the skeleton including extremities
18. mineral stored by the bones
20. inward curve of the cervical and lumbar areas of the spine

Developing Vocabulary

Writing Practice

Beside each word below, write a complete sentence using the word. For each sentence, check for accuracy of content, spelling, and punctuation.

1. axial ____

____

____

2. articulation _____________________________________

____

____

3. gout ____

____

____

4. joints ____

____

____

5. etiology ____

____

____

6. concave ____

____

____

7. epiphysis ____

____

____

8. ligament ____

____

____

True or False

If the definition on the right corresponds to the word on the left, then check True; if the word and definition do not correspond, check False.

TRUE	FALSE	WORD
____	____	1. **Lordosis:** bone tissue that is spongy and porous
____	____	2. **Fractures:** broken bones
____	____	3. **Bone spurs:** growths of excess bone along joint edges
____	____	4. **Diaphysis:** the central shaft of the long bones
____	____	5. **Axial:** sideway curvature of any section of the vertebral spine

Spell Correctly

In each of the sets of words below, one word is spelled correctly. Circle the correctly spelled word.

1.
   a. scolisois
   b. scociosis
   c. scoliosis
   d. scolcosis

2.
   a. inturvertebral
   b. intervertebral
   c. interverteiral
   d. intervertebrul

3.
   a. osteopotosis
   b. osteoporosis
   c. ostetporosis
   d. ostioporosis

4.
   a. rhuematoid
   b. rmeumatoid
   c. rheumatiid
   d. rheumatoid

5.
   a. cartilege
   b. carsilage
   c. cartigage
   d. cartilage

Practice Scenario(s)

After reading this chapter in the text, read the following scenario(s) and answer the questions following each of them.

Situation 1

You are assigned to assist a patient with ambulation (walking), and you noticed that he is limping. He seems to be protecting the right leg, bearing more weight on the left side.

1. What should you do?

____

____

____

Situation 2

You are assigned to assist a patient with ambulation, and she uses a cane.

1. What is the correct procedure for assisting this patient?

____

____

____

Situation 3

You are assigned to Mr. Abdul, who is unable to move or stand without assistance because he has had a stroke. The stroke affected his left leg, causing severe weakness. He spends much of his day immobile, remaining in bed or in a lounge chair.

1. What can you do to provide weight bearing activity for Mr. Abdul?

____

____

____

Situation 4

Mrs. Cammarota has had a stroke, which affected the left side of her body. She has been admitted to your long-term care facility for rehabilitation. She has weakness of the left arm and leg and needs assistance with activities of daily living (ADLs). She is left-handed.

1. With which ADLs will Mrs. Cammarota require your assistance?

____

____

____

The Muscular System

Chapter Review

Multiple Choice

1. Which type of muscle is controlled voluntarily?
   a. smooth
   c. striated
   b. visceral
   d. branching

2. Visceral muscle tissues move all except
   a. food.
   c. blood.
   b. urine.
   d. bones.

3. The end of the muscle that is attached to the stationary bone is called the
   a. origin.
   c. insertion.
   b. ligament.
   d. isometric.

4. The muscle that is responsible for flexion of the forearm is the
   a. biceps.
   b. triceps.
   c. deltoid.
   d. trapezius.

5. Movement toward the midline of the body is called
   a. abduction.
   b. obliteration.
   c. adduction.
   d. flexion.

6. Which muscle is NOT used for I.M. injections?
   a. sternocleidomastoid
   b. deltoid
   c. gluteus medius
   d. vastus lateralis

7. Which type of muscle tissue is found in blood vessels and internal organs of the digestive and urinary systems?
   a. smooth and cardiac
   b. smooth and visceral
   c. striated and visceral
   d. branching and visceral

8. Which type of muscle tissue works every second of an individual's life?
   a. branching, smooth
   b. cardiac, smooth
   c. skeletal, smooth
   d. cardiac, branching

9. What condition results when muscle fibers shorten and remain in a fixed position?
   a. dysplasia
   b. hypertrophy
   c. contracture
   d. infarction

10. Atrophy is
    a. shrinking or deterioration of muscle tissue.
    b. overdevelopment of muscle tissue.
    c. shortening and thickening of muscles.
    d. painful abduction of muscle tissues.

11. The large muscles of the anterior surface of the thigh are collectively called
    a. hamstrings.   c. quadriceps.
    b. abductors.   d. triceps.

12. What is necessary for healthy muscle tone?
    a. rest   c. exercise
    b. flexion   d. vitamin D

13. The CCA's observation of the client's skeletal muscle would include all but
    a. the ability to walk
    b. mobility in bed
    c. performance of ADL's
    d. digestion of food

14. The inability to move or to feel the body from the waist to the toes is called
    a. hemiplegia.
    b. paraplegia.
    c. quadriplegia.
    d. totoplegia.

Identification Exercise

Label the figure below:

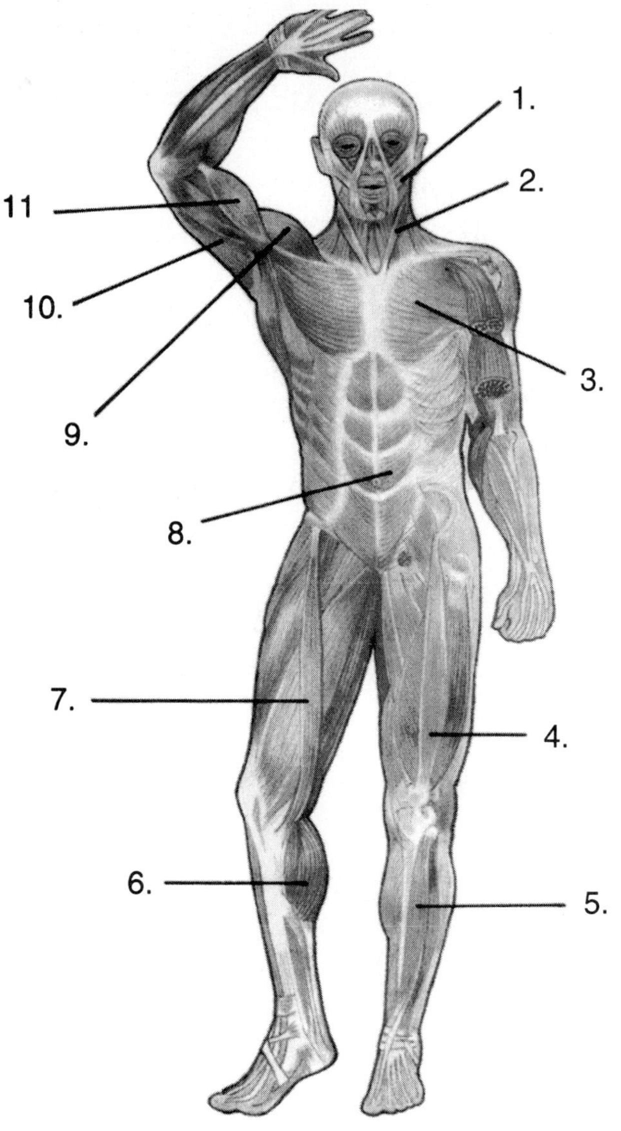

1._______________________   7._______________________

2._______________________   8._______________________

3._______________________   9._______________________

4._______________________   10._______________________

5._______________________   11._______________________

6._______________________

Vocabulary Activity

The following word search puzzle contains terms that are found in this chapter. Use the word list below to locate the hidden words in the grid.

```
O G N T G Z W K B I M M Z Q D X R L R G
M U W J T M F R S S M J D E N J N N B Z
T H N V M Y P J V O L U N T A R Y U I J
I D S S V N A W F M R O H S R J W Y F B
L S M J I A B V T E N D O N S C B N X I
J D O L E Y D Q K T I Y N A D E A K B A
I B O T Z F U D R R D J L R T K X E E F
U I T A O I C X U I X Z P F O I Z Q I F
U X H V B N T S N C N B A J N Q C X N P
F I I E M X I B T U T I W L G R O T C I
C O O K M Y O C A R D I U M O R D U Q W
R Z M T E I N P X L I H O Q K D K Y J T
A B P A R A P L E G I A D N S E J F E A
M L H T D E N L G A P A T R O P H Y Z G
J C Z V A L F L E X I O N E W B U G P U
T S H N B N F B O G G P U G D I J A U K
T D M I N F A R C T I O N M E Z A U A Q
Q U A D R I P L E G I A S S H G I Z V V
J C C K I M E E J Q B Y C E L X W A O
D T Z P M J M I Y A S X U V W N T Q F K
```

1. abduction
2. adduction
3. atrophy
4. flexion
5. hemiplegia
6. infarction
7. isometric
8. isotonic
9. myocardium
10. paraplegia
11. quadriplegia
12. smooth
13. striated
14. tendons
15. voluntary

Developing Vocabulary

Writing Practice

Beside each word below, write a complete sentence using the word. For each sentence, check for accuracy of content, spelling, and punctuation.

1. smooth ____

____

____

2. extension ____

____

____

3. adduction ____

____

____

4. hypertrophy ______________________________________

____

____

5. insertion ____

____

____

6. involuntary _______________________________________

____

____

7. myasthenia _______________________________________

____

____

8. paralysis____

____

____

True or False

If the definition on the right corresponds to the word on the left, then check True, if the word and definition do not correspond, check False.

TRUE	FALSE	WORD
____	____	1. **Voluntary:** muscle contraction that generates movement
____	____	2. **Hemiplegia:** paralysis of one side of the body
____	____	3. **Flexion:** movement decreasing the angle of a joint
____	____	4. **Tendons:** attachment between bone and muscle
____	____	5. **Isotonic:** paralysis of the lower extremities

Spell Correctly

In each of the sets of words below, one word is spelled correctly. Circle the correctly spelled word.

1. a. quadrillegia   c. quadriplegia
    b. qudariplegia   d. quadrodplegia

2. a. abduction   c. abductaon
    b. abducsion   d. abductoin

3. a. struated   c. straited
    b. striated   d. staiated

4. a. isometrrc   c. isometric
    b. isomatric   d. isometrec

5. a. myocarduim   c. myocardeum
    b. myocardium   d. myocardoum

Practice Scenario(s)

After reading this chapter in the text, read the following scenario(s) and answer the questions following each of them.

Situation 1

Mrs. Grace has suffered a stroke, and you are assigned to provide physical care for her. She was admitted to the hospital two days ago, and the stroke has affected her right side. As you begin to assist her with her bed bath, you see that her right hand is bent back and is fixed in this position.

1. What do you do?

____

____

____

Situation 2

Mr. Sherone is a 40-year-old man who was in a car accident and has had injury to his spinal cord at L4 (lumbar vertebra # 4). As a result of this injury, he has paraplegia. He was admitted to your rehabilitation unit yesterday. The first goal he has set with his physical therapist is to learn to transfer himself from bed to wheelchair. Mr. Sherone was in the spinal cord unit at the university hospital for three weeks. Today, he will begin to learn this transfer technique. The nurse tells you that Mr.Sherone will need assistance with his ADLs and encouragement in performing active ROM exercises of the upper extremities and passive ROM to the lower extremities. He is on a bowel retraining program.

1. How will you plan to proceed with your A.M.care?

____

____

____

2. What do the nurse's instructions mean to you?

____

____

____

Situation 3

Mr. Sherone has been your patient for three days, and you notice that the pressure ulcer on his coccyx has progressed from a stage one to a stage two. Ever since the physical therapist has taught him to transfer from bed to chair, he has remained OOB for at least four hours at a time. You know that he should not remain in one position for more than two hours, but he seems so much happier when he is OOB in his wheelchair and roaming about the rehab unit. You want to promote this independence, and you want to see him happy. Mr. Sherone has not worn anything on his feet except his soft slippers since he arrived on your unit. He says, "My feet don't work, and I feel stupid wearing shoes."

1. What will you do?

____

____

____

Situation 4

You are assigned to Mrs. Polaski, and you are informed by the nurse that you are to perform passive ROM exercises to all extremities. Mrs. Polaski has myasthenia gravis, is very weak, and tires easily. One day you are performing an exercise that moves the arms away from the midline of the body, and she screams in pain when you abduct the left arm.

1. What do you do?

____

____

____

Chapter 10

The Nervous System

Chapter Review

Multiple Choice

1. The basic structure or unit of the nervous system is the
   a. neuroma.
   b. schwann cell.
   c. neurolemma.
   d. neuron.

2. Which part of the nerve cell conducts messages to the cell body?
   a. axon
   b. dendrite
   c. myelin sheath
   d. schwann cell

3. Which type of neuron directs signals to the brain and spinal cord?
   a. interneuron
   b. motor neuron
   c. sensory neuron
   d. neurolemma

4. Interneurons
   a. are found only in the spinal cord.
   b. connect messages from the brain to the spinal cord.
   c. are found only in the ANS.
   d. relay messages from spinal nerves to cranial nerves.

5. The organs of the CNS include
   a. brain and ANS.
   b. brain and spinal nerves.
   c. PNS and ANS.
   d. brain and spinal cord.

6. The largest section of the human brain is the
   a. cerebellum.
   b. midbrain.
   c. cerebrum.
   d. thalamus.

7. Which lobe of the cerebrum controls movement of the left arm and leg?
   a. left occipital
   b. right temporal
   c. left parietal
   d. right frontal

8. The area of the brain responsible for reflex functions of respiration, heart rate, and blood pressure is the
   a. pons.
   b. medulla oblongata.
   c. hypothalamus.
   d. cerebellum.

9. The relay center for sensory information and direction of sensory messages in the brain is the
   a. hypothalamus.
   b. cerebrum.
   c. thalamus.
   d. cerebellum.

10. Which area of the brain controls appetite, body temperature, thirst, and the pituitary gland's release of hormones?
    a. hypothalamus
    b. thalamus
    c. cerebrum
    d. cerebellum

11. The colored part of the eye is the
    a. retina.
    b. sclera.
    c. lens.
    d. pupil.

12. The part of the eye that contains receptors for day and night vision is the
    a. lens.
    b. cornea.
    c. retina.
    d. pupil.

13. The division of the ANS that is concerned with controlling the body's responses to stress is
    a. parasympathetic.
    b. paraplegia.
    c. sympathetic.
    d. cholinergic.

14. Causes of a CVA include all except
    a. thrombus.
    b. hemorrhage.
    c. embolus.
    d. calculi

Identification Exercise

Label the figure below:

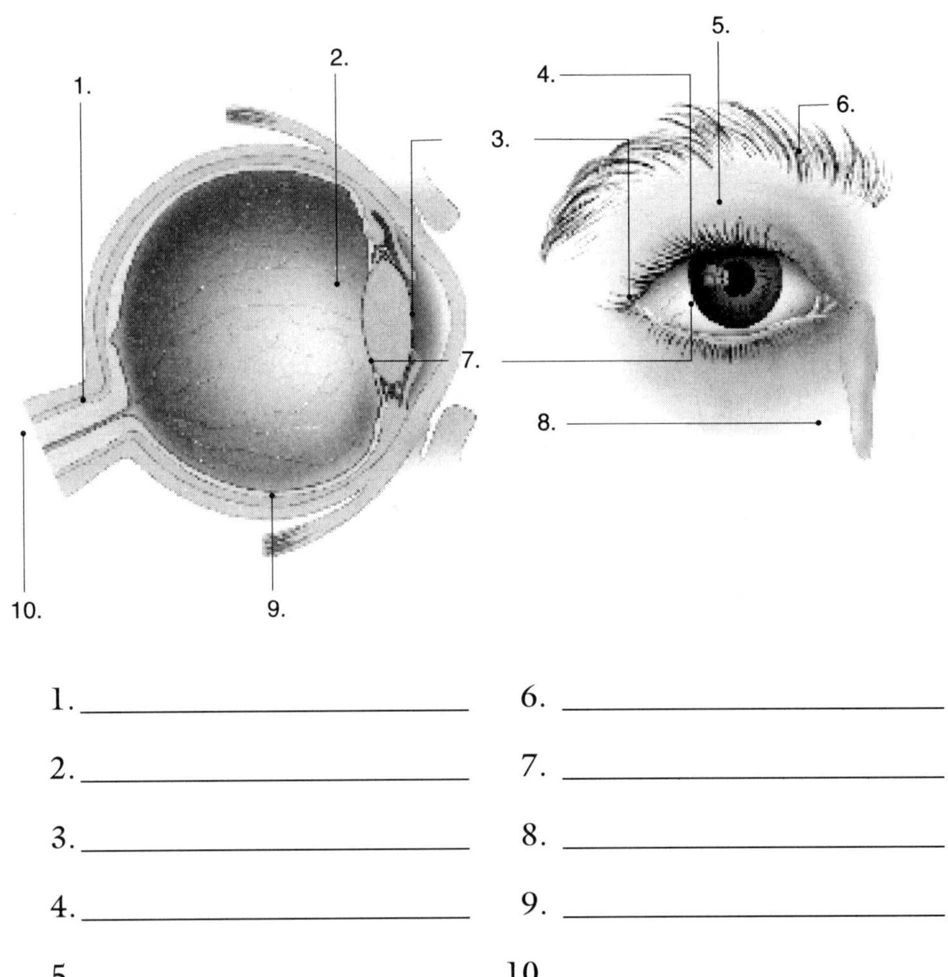

1. _______________________

2. _______________________

3. _______________________

4. _______________________

5. _______________________

6. _______________________

7. _______________________

8. _______________________

9. _______________________

10. _______________________

Vocabulary Activity

The following crossword puzzle contains terms that are found in this chapter. Use the clues below to complete the puzzle.

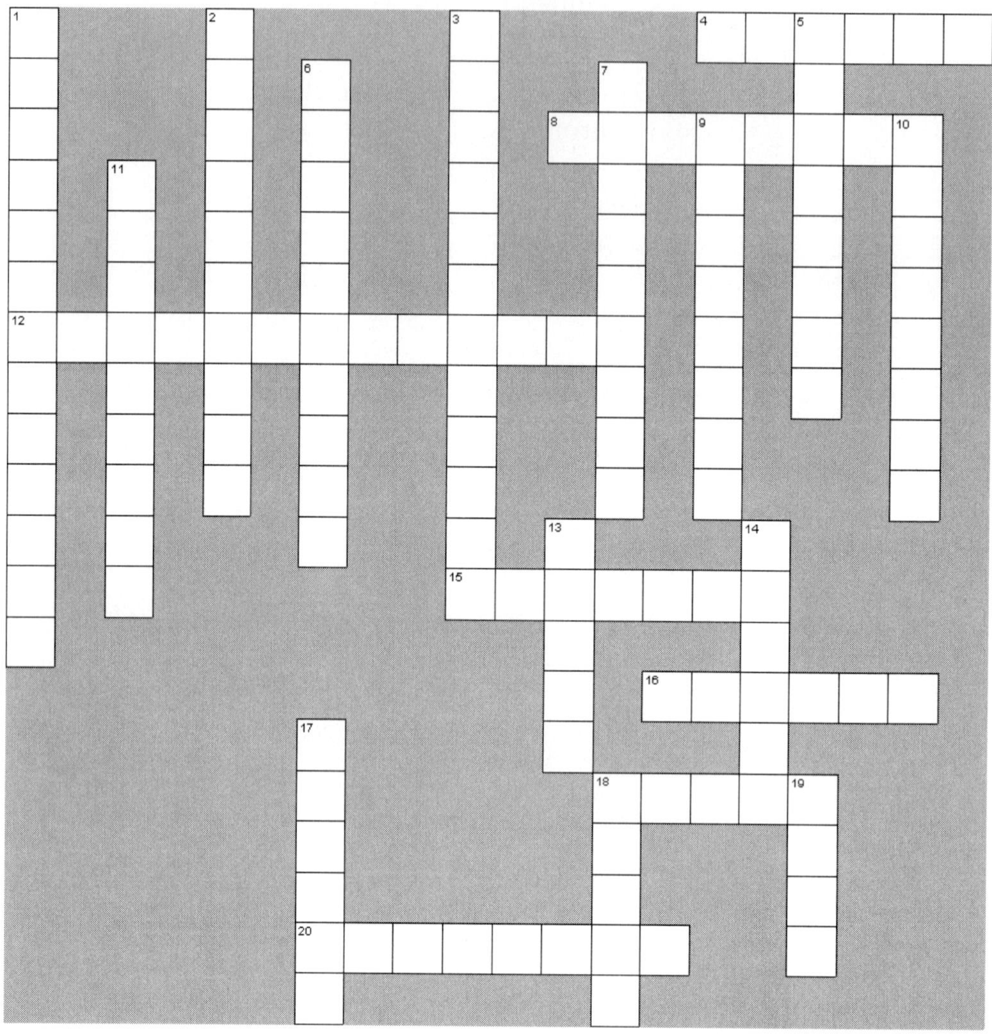

ACROSS

4. innermost vascular layer of the eye
8. largest section of brain responsible for thought, reason, creativity, and feelings
12. grossly enlarged head resulting from obstructed flow of cerebrospinal fluid
15. juncture between two neurons
16. cerebrovascular accident
18. visible part of the external ear
20. reflex center resting atop the pons, responsible for hearing and eye movements

DOWN

1. protein substance that sends a message
2. loss of accommodation; old age vision
3. part of the brain responsible for unconscious and autonomic control
5. blood clot that forms in a blood vessel
6. part of the brain that controls balance
7. temporary disappearance of symptoms
9. seizure disorder of unknown origin, with seizure the primary symptom
10. protective membrane that covers the brain and spinal cord
11. part of the neuron that conducts messages to the cell body
13. one of the middle ear bones that vibrates to transmit sound
14. nerve cell
17. tumor of the glial cells, a type of brain cell
18. open area in the center of the iris that adjusts the amount of light entering the eye
19. part of the neuron that conducts messages away from the cell body

Developing Vocabulary

Writing Practice

Beside each word below, write a complete sentence using the word. For each sentence, check for accuracy of content, spelling, and punctuation.

1. midbrain ____

\
____

2. neurochemical ____

\
____

3. remission ____

\
____

4. axon ____

\
____

5. cerebellum ____

\
____

6. glioma ____

\
____

7. pinna ____

\
____

8. incus ____

\
____

True/False

If the definition on the right corresponds to the word on the left, then check True, if the word and definition do not correspond, check False.

TRUE	FALSE	WORD
____	____	1. **Retina:** the innermost vascular layer of the eye
____	____	2. **Stroke:** protective membrane that covers the brain and spinal cord
____	____	3. **Pupil:** nerve cell
____	____	4. **Meninges:** cerebrovascular accident
____	____	5. **Epilepsy:** seizure disorder of unknown origin with seizures the primary symptom

Spell Correctly

In each of the sets of words below, one word is spelled correctly. Circle the correctly spelled word.

1.
   a. hydrhcephalus
   b. hydrocephalus
   c. hydrecephalus
   d. hydrocephulus

2.
   a. glimo
   b. gliima
   c. glioma
   d. gloima

3.
   a. hypothalamos
   b. hypothalamus
   c. hypothplamus
   d. hypothalemus

4.
   a. presbyopua
   b. presbyopea
   c. presbyopia
   d. prosbyopia

5.
   a. synepse
   b. synapse
   c. sysapse
   d. synupse

Practice Scenario(s)

After reading this chapter in the text, read the following scenario(s) and answer the questions following each of them.

Situation 1

Miss Jones is 17 years old. She was admitted to your pediatric unit last night following a car accident. She suffered a skull fracture that did not lacerate the brain. You are assigned to care for her, and the nurse's report reveals the following information. She is complaining of a headache, dizziness, and nausea. She is able to speak and to voluntarily move her limbs, and she has not lost consciousness. She is NPO (nothing by mouth) until 12 noon and on bedrest. You are to observe her for signs of neurological changes and to assist her with A.M. care. Upon entering her room, you see that she is getting out of her bed. She tells you that she has to go to the bathroom to use the toilet and to get a drink of water.

1. Describe how you will proceed.

____

____

____

Situation 2

Mr. Weatherby is a 68-year-old man who was admitted to the emergency room (ER) two hours ago. When you arrive, you get a report about Mr. Weatherby. The nurse tells you that he had a CVA. A computerized axial tomography (CAT) scan revealed a blood clot in the left frontal lobe.

1. What impairments do you expect he will have?

____

____

____

Situation 3

Mrs. Gabet is a 42-year-old woman who has a glioma (tumor of the glial cells of the brain) in the right occipital lobe. She is being admitted to your oncology unit for chemotherapy and radiation. You are to orient her to her room, take her vital signs, chart her height and weight, and complete the inventory of her belongings.

1. What symptoms do you expect Mrs. Gabet to have, and what assistance do you think you will need to give her?

____

____

____

Situation 4

Bobby Esposito is a 6-year-old boy who fell last week while riding his bike. His mother has brought him to the doctor's office for a checkup because of complaints of a headache and excessive sleeping. Yesterday, he came home from school with a bruise over his left eye, and he does not remember how he got it. As you enter the exam room to take his vital signs, you hear him cry out. He falls to the ground and begins to have jerking movements of the limbs. He arches his back, and you see frothy saliva coming out of his mouth.

1. What do you do?

____

____

____

C h a p t e r 1 1

The Circulatory System

Chapter Review

Multiple Choice

1. Blood vessels transport all but
   a. hormones.
   b. nutrients.
   c. waste products.
   d. lymph.

2. The muscular layer of the heart is called the
   a. pericardium.
   b. myocardium.
   c. epicardium.
   d. endocardium.

3. The heart has __________ chambers.
   a. two
   b. three
   c. four
   d. five

4. Blood is emptied into the left atrium by way of the
   a. aorta.
   b. vena cava.
   c. pulmonary vein.
   d. coronary artery.

5. The chamber of the heart that pumps oxygenated blood to the
   aorta is the
   a. right ventricle.
   b. left ventricle.
   c. left atrium.
   d. right atrium.

6. The _________ valve lies between the left atrium and the left ventricle.
    a. pulmonic
    b. aortic
    c. tricuspid
    d. bicuspid

7. The _________ valve lies between the right atrium and the right ventricle.
    a. tricuspid
    b. bicuspid
    c. pulmonic
    d. aortic

8. The blood vessels that supply the heart with nutrients and oxygen are the _________ arteries.
    a. carotid
    b. myocardial
    c. coronary
    d. pulmonary

9. What sets the pace for the heart's rate and rhythm?
    a. bundle of His
    b. Purkinje fibers
    c. sinoatrial node
    d. atrioventricular node

10. Which blood vessel carries oxygenated blood exclusively?
    a. artery
    b. vein
    c. capillaries
    d. lymph

11. Which type of blood cell protects the body against infection?
    a. karyocyte
    b. erythrocyte
    c. leukocyte
    d. thrombocyte

12. When measuring a patient's pulse, which characteristic are you noting?
    a. rate
    b. rhythm
    c. force
    d. volume

13. Which lymph organ destroys old RBC's and stores blood?
    a. tonsil
    b. thymus
    c. node
    d. spleen

14. The accessory organs of the lymphatic system include all of the following except
    a. tonsils.
    b. thymus.
    c. spleen.
    d. liver.

15. Red blood cells carry __________ on the hemoglobin molecule.
    a. oxygen
    b. carbon dioxide
    c. glucose
    d. albumin

Identification Exercise

Label the figure on the following page:

1. __________________________   8. __________________________

2. __________________________   9. __________________________

3. __________________________   10. _________________________

4. __________________________   11. _________________________

5. __________________________   12. _________________________

6. __________________________   13. _________________________

7. __________________________

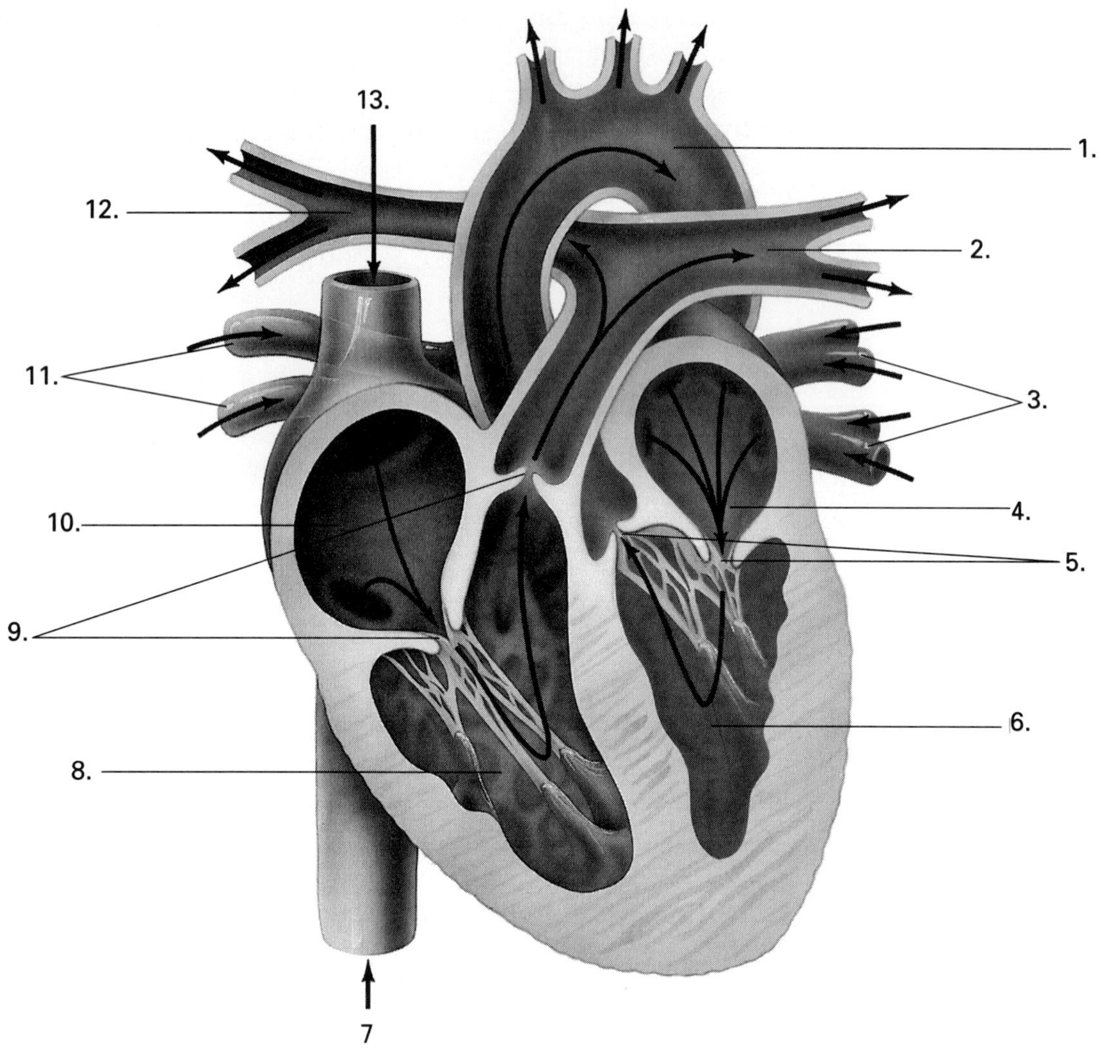

Vocabulary Activity

The following crossword puzzle contains terms that are found in this chapter. Use the clues below to complete the puzzle.

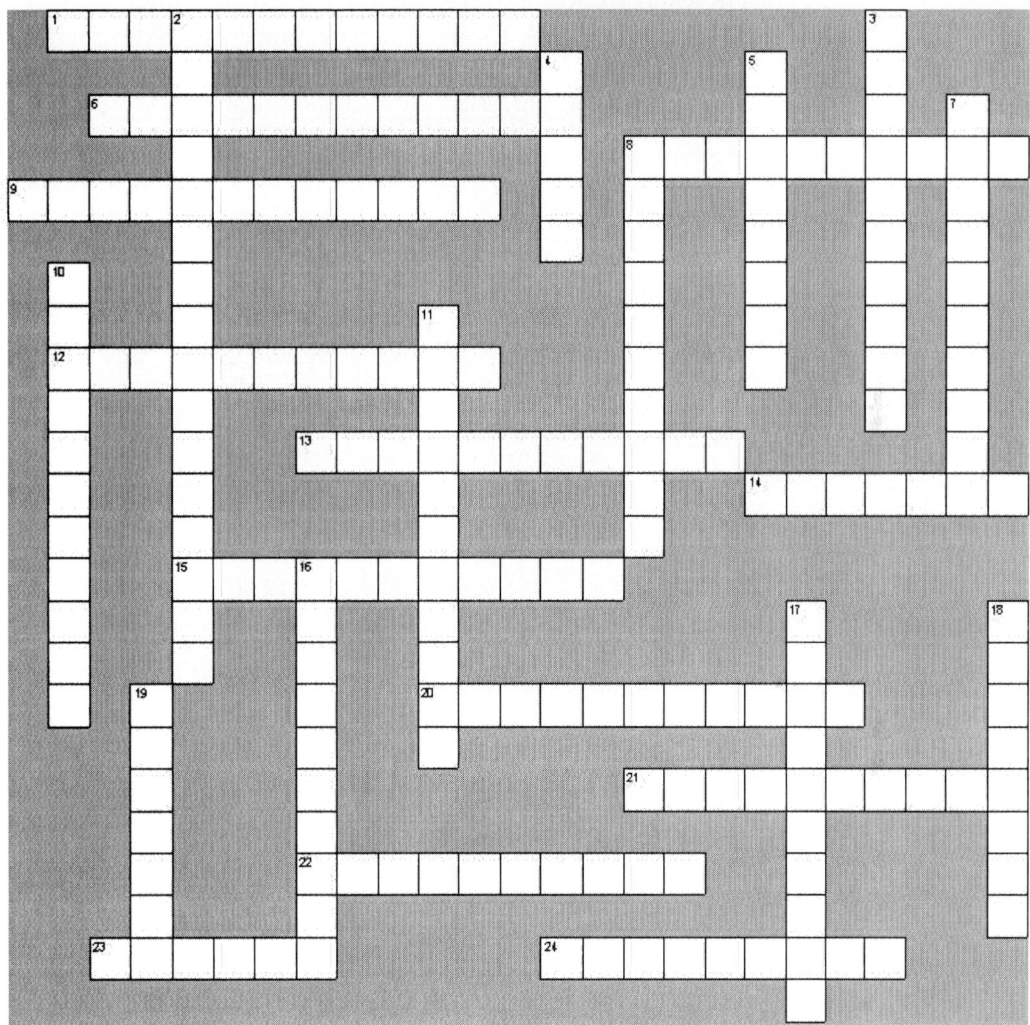

ACROSS

1. red blood cells
6. abnormally enlarged heart
8. small arteries
9. clotting cells
12. deviation from normal heartbeat pattern
13. fibroserous sac around the heart
14. substance that, when detected in the body, causes formation of an antibody
15. abnormally fast heart rate over 100 beats per minute
20. inner heart layer
21. type of white blood cell that digests microbes and cellular debris
22. white blood cells
23. chest pain
24. broad category of simple proteins

DOWN

2. inflammation of the vein due to blood clot
3. complex protein–iron compound that carries oxygen to the cells
4. thin fluid originating in organs and tissues
5. localized dilation and subsequent thinning of a blood vessel wall
7. device for separating blood into liquid and solids
8. immunoglobulin essential to the immune system
10. heart rate less than 60 beats per minute
11. thin wall, tiny blood vessels at the arteriovenous junction
16. hereditary bleeding disorder in which there is a deficiency of one of the clotting factors
17. decrease number of white cells
18. having two points or cusps in relation to the mitral valve
19. blood protein

Developing Vocabulary

Writing Practice

Beside each word below, write a complete sentence using the word. For each sentence, check for accuracy of content, spelling, and punctuation.

1. aneurysm ____

    ____

    ____

2. endocardium ____

    ____

    ____

3. angina ____

    ____

    ____

4. centrifuge ____

    ____

    ____

5. pericardium ____

    ____

    ____

6. leukocytes ____

    ____

    ____

7. arrhythmias ____

    ____

    ____

8. hemophilia ____

    ____

    ____

True or False

If the definition on the right corresponds to the word on the left, then check True, if the word and definition do not correspond, check False.

TRUE   FALSE   WORD

____   ____   1. **Globulins:** substance that, when detected in the body, causes formation of an antibody

____   ____   2. **Antibodies:** immunoglobulin essential to the immune system

____   ____   3. **Phagocytes:** type of white blood cell that digests microbes and cellular debris

____   ____   4. **Antigen:** hereditary bleeding disorder in which there is a deficiency of one of the clotting factors

____   ____   5. **Tachycardia:** abnormally fast heart rate over 100 beats per minute

Spell Correctly

In each of the sets of words below, one word is spelled correctly. Circle the correctly spelled word.

1.   a. artorioles   c. arteriales
       b. arteriolus   d. arterioles

2.   a. erythrecytes   c. eyythrocytes
       b. ersthrocytes   d. erythrocytes

3.   a. thrombophlibitis   c. thrombophiebitis
       b. thrombophlebitis   d. thromrophlebitis

4.   a. leukopenia   c. leukoeenia
       b. leukepenia   d. llukopenia

5.   a. bradycardia   c. bradicardia
       b. bradycardea   d. bridycardia

Practice Scenario(s)

After reading this chapter in the text, read the following scenario(s) and answer the questions following each of them.

Situation 1

Mrs. O'Maley is a 42-year-old woman who was admitted to the CCU yesterday. She arrived in the ER with complaints of dizziness, palpitations, and sweating when she was doing her morning exercises. She was found to have an irregular ECG with multiple premature ventricular contractions (PVCs) and ventricular tachycardia.

1. What is your understanding of Ventricular Tachycardia?

2. What test was used to detect this condition?

3. How will Mrs. O'Maley's heart status be monitored in the C.C.U.?

Situation 2

Mr. Vegas is a 76-year-old man and a resident in the LTC facility. You have known him for a year. His diagnosis is CHF. He is sometimes short of breath, and you know he takes a medication for his heart. The nurse always reminds you to take his pulse before the 8:00 A.M. medication is given. When you enter his room at 7:30 A.M., he is sitting in a chair, and his breathing is labored. When you look at his feet, you see that they are puffy, and his slippers are too tight for his feet. You take his vital signs, and these are your findings: pulse 106, respirations 34, blood pressure 168/102, temperature 98.4°F.

1. What will you report to the nurse, and when will you report these findings?

____

____

____

2. Which of Mr. Vegas's vital signs are abnormal, or out of normal range?

____

____

____

3. Why are Mr. Vegas's feet swollen?

____

____

____

4. Why is Mr. Vegas's breathing loud and labored?

____

____

____

Situation 3

Mr. Smythe is a 22-year-old with a diagnosis of acute leukemia. He is admitted to the oncology unit for chemotherapy and is placed on neutropenic precautions. The sign on Mr. Smythe's door reads *NEU-TROPENIC PRECAUTIONS: Anyone who enters must wear a mask. Do not bring fresh fruits or flowers into the room.*

1. Why is Mr. Smythe placed on neutropenic precautions?

____

____

____

2. Why does the sign on the door have warnings about fresh fruits and fresh flowers?

____

____

____

Situation 4

Ms. Le is a 10-year-old patient. She was in an auto accident and was admitted to the trauma unit at the university hospital. She is receiving blood transfusions because she had multiple injuries that resulted in hemorrhage. You heard the physician say that she had a lacerated spleen. One of your duties is to pick up blood products from the blood bank. The first time you are sent you pick up a pint of whole blood identified as B+. A few hours later you are asked to get a unit of packed cells. At 9:00 P.M. you are asked to take Ms. Le's vital signs before the nurse hangs the blood and to check them again 5 minutes and 15 minutes after the transfusion is started. The nurse hangs the blood at 9:10 pm. These are your results at 9:15 P.M.: 99.4°F, 122-30, BP-72/44.

1. Does the injury to Ms. Le's spleen have anything to do with the hemorrhage?

____

____

____

2. What does the B+ blood indicate to you about Ms. Le's blood type?

____

____

____

3. What is the difference between the unit of whole blood and the unit of packed cells?

____

____

____

4. Why are Ms. Le's pulse and respirations so rapid and her blood pressure so low?

____

____

____

Situation 5

Mr. Byrd is a 70-year-old patient admitted to the hospital for abdominal surgery. He is two days postop and is receiving an antibiotic medication intravenously. The IV is in his left lower arm. As you are assisting him with A.M. care, he complains of pain at the IV site. You look at the IV site and note that it is red and swollen; it feels warm to the touch.

1. What should you do and why?

____

____

____

Situation 6

Mr. Nyugen is 45-year-old man who arrives at the ER complaining of weakness and shortness of breath. He is admitted to the ER and, while you are taking his vital signs and waiting for the nurse to assess him, he complains of severe chest pain. His pulse is weak, rapid, and irregular. He is sweating and pale.

1. What do you do?

____

____

____

The Respiratory System

Chapter Review

Multiple Choice

1. External respiration is accomplished in the
   a. lungs.
   b. cells of the body.
   c. bronchi.
   d. capillaries.

2. The respiratory system helps to balance the pH of blood by removing __________ from the blood.
   a. oxygen
   b. carbon dioxide
   c. water
   d. hydrochloric acid

3. Which of the following is an organ of the digestive and respiratory systems?
   a. larynx
   b. trachea
   c. esophagus
   d. pharynx

4. The range of normal blood pH is
   a. 5.4–5.5.
   b. 7.1–7.6.
   c. 7.35–7.45.
   d. 7.2–7.7.

5. Inflammation of the lining of the thoracic cavity is called
   a. thoracocentesis.
   b. pleurisy.
   c. pleural edema.
   d. pneumonitis.

6. The voice box is the
   a. pharynx.
   b. trachea.
   c. bronchi.
   d. larynx.

7. While swallowing food, the __________ protects the larynx from aspiration
   a. thyroid
   b. vocal cords
   c. glottis
   d. epiglottis

8. The __________ are microscopic structures that exchange oxygen and carbon dioxide with capillaries in the lungs.
   a. pleural sacs
   b. alveoli
   c. bronchioles
   d. capillary sacs

9. The rate and depth of respirations are regulated by the
   a. medulla oblongata.
   b. lungs.
   c. cerebellum.
   d. thalamus.

10. Which of the following is NOT true about asthma?
   a. May be caused by food allergies
   b. A condition of intermittent obstruction of bronchial tubes
   c. Symptoms include rales and prolonged inspiration
   d. Symptoms include wheezing and prolonged expiration

11. COPD is a general term used to describe all except
   a. chronic lung conditions.
   b. chronic bronchitis.
   c. emphysema.
   d. pulmonary edema.

12. An infectious disease of the lungs caused by a bacteria is
   a. asthma.
   b. emphysema.
   c. tuberculosis.
   d. AIDS.

13. When a hospitalized patient has active TB, the patient is placed in __________ isolation.
   a. droplet
   b. contact
   c. reverse
   d. airborne

14. The term that describes difficult breathing is
   a. tachypnea.
   b. dyspnea.
   c. apnea.
   d. bradypnea.

Identification Exercise

Label the figure on the following page:

1._______________________	10. _______________________
2._______________________	11. _______________________
3._______________________	12. _______________________
4._______________________	13. _______________________
5._______________________	14. _______________________
6._______________________	15. _______________________
7._______________________	16. _______________________
8._______________________	17. _______________________
9._______________________	

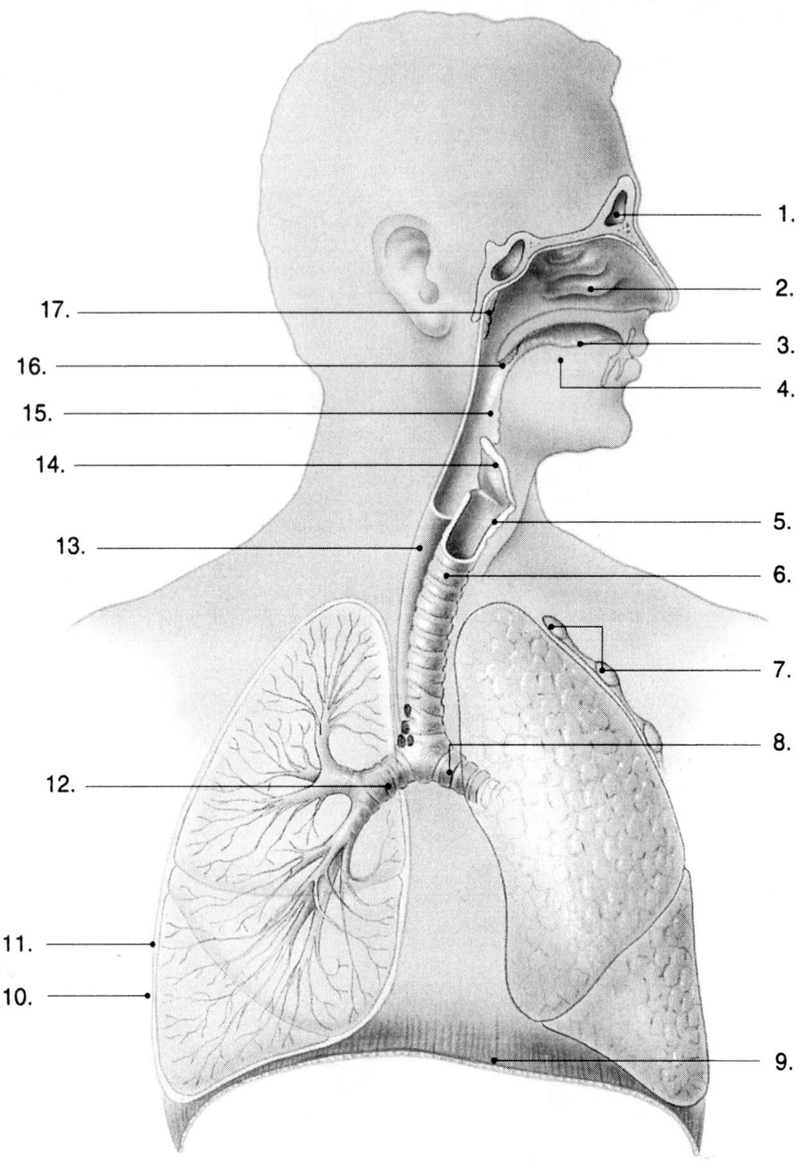
1.
2.
3.
4.
5.
6.
7.
8.
9.
10.
11.
12.
13.
14.
15.
16.
17.

Vocabulary Activity

The following crossword puzzle contains terms that are found in this chapter. Use the clues below to complete the puzzle.

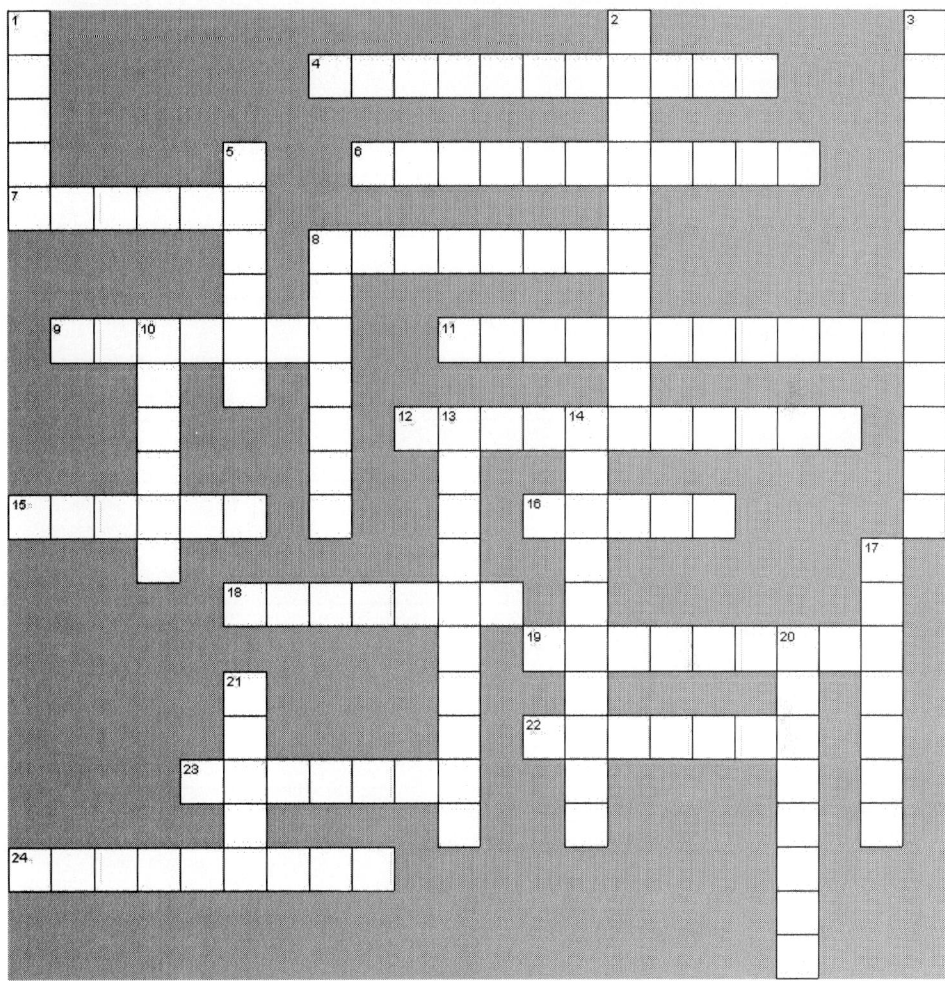

ACROSS

4. small passageways extending from the bronchi
6. process of inhaling and exhaling
7. intermittent construction of the bronchial tubes
8. pertaining to the chest cavity
9. difficulty breathing
11. infectious disease of the lungs caused by a bacteria, a tubercle bacillus
12. center of the thorax
15. protective membrane of the thoracic cavity
16. without breathing
18. small air sacs located at the base of the lungs
19. rapid breathing
22. cavities in the head and face bones
23. major passageways to lungs
24. disease resulting from chronic inflammatory and obstructive conditions of the lungs

DOWN

1. tiny hairlike structures lining the nose
2. fibrous bands in the larynx responsible for speech
3. creation of a new opening into the trachea to bypass the upper respiratory tree
5. voice box
8. windpipe
10. wall or partition that forms the right and left nostrils
13. cartilage that closes off the larynx when swallowing
14. act of breathing in vomitus or object in the throat into the lungs
17. throat
20. openings to the hose divided by the septum
21. synonym for nostrils

Developing Vocabulary

Writing Practice

Beside each word below, write a complete sentence using the word. For each sentence, check for accuracy of content, spelling, and punctuation.

1. apnea ____

    ____

    ____

2. nostrils ____

    ____

    ____

3. septum ____

    ____

    ____

4. aspiration ____

    ____

    ____

5. thoracic ____

    ____

    ____

6. mediastinum ____

    ____

    ____

7. bronchioles ____

    ____

    ____

8. trachea ____

    ____

    ____

True or False

If the definition on the right corresponds to the word on the left, then check True; if the word and definition do not correspond, check False.

TRUE   FALSE   WORD

____   ____   1. **Tachypnea:** difficulty breathing

____   ____   2. **Tuberculosis:** infectious disease of the lungs caused by a bacteria, a tubercle bacillus

____   ____   3. **Emphysema:** disease resulting from chronic inflammatory and obstructive conditions of the lungs

____   ____   4. **Sinuses:** openings to the nose divided by the septum

____   ____   5. **Tracheostomy:** creation of a new opening into the trachea to bypass the upper respiratory tree

Spell Correctly

In each of the sets of words below, one word is spelled correctly. Circle the correctly spelled word.

1.   a. cilaa   c. cilea
      b. cilia   d. celia

2.   a. bronchi   c. brenchi
      b. brbnchi   d. brinchi

3.   a. tuuerculosis   c. tubreculosis
      b. tubercusosis   d. tuberculosis

4.   a. emphysima   c. emphysama
      b. emphysema   d. esphysema

5.   a. nostnils   c. nostrils
      b. nostrols   d. nistrils

Practice Scenario(s)

After reading this chapter in the text, read the following scenario(s) and answer the questions following each of them.

Situation 1

You are feeding a patient breakfast, and the patient begins to talk as he is chewing his toast. Suddenly, the patient chokes, and his face turns bright red.

1. What actions will you take?

____

____

____

Situation 2

Mrs. Cruz is a 70-year-old woman who has been admitted to the orthopedic unit following a left hip replacement. She is receiving 4L O_2 via a mask. You are assigned to assist her with care two days post-op. When you enter the room, you see that she is washing her face and has removed the O_2 mask. Your first interventions involve taking vital signs. As you speak with her, you notice that she is short of breath and that she looks pale and sweaty. Her temperature is normal, but her pulse is rapid 106, respirations 34, and blood pressure (BP) 160/90.

1. What is your immediate action?

____

____

____

Situation 3

Two days later, Mrs. Cruz returns to your unit from the intensive care unit (ICU). You are assigned to Mrs. Cruz again. Today, you are told that she had pulmonary embolism and that she is now receiving O_2 at 6L and intravenous heparin, an anticoagulant.

1. What do you think these treatment changes indicate?

____

____

____

Situation 4

Mr. Augustin is a 40-year-old man who is being admitted to your
unit today. He has a diagnosis of AIDS and rule out (r/o) TB. You
are assigned to set up his room. The unit clerk tells you he is assigned
to isolation room 102.

1. Why does he have a special isolation room?

____

____

____

2. What supplies do you need to prepare for his admission?

____

____

____

Situation 5

Mr. Augustin asks you why his door remains closed and why you are
wearing a mask when you enter his room.

1. What do you tell him?

____

____

____

2. What special instructions does he need regarding (r/o) TB?

____

____

____

Situation 6

Mrs. Ramos is a patient in your rehabilitation unit. She was admitted
following treatment in the hospital for multiple injuries from a
MVA (motor vehicle accident). Today is the first day that you have
been assigned to her. She has had a tracheostomy because of damage

to her trachea from the crash. You have never had a patient with a tracheostomy.

1. What do you expect to find when you meet Mrs. Ramos?

____

____

____

Situation 7

Jenny Smith is a 12-year-old girl who had abdominal surgery two days ago. You are told in report to encourage her to cough and deep-breathe and to use the incentive spirometer.

1. Why?

____

____

____

The Digestive System

Chapter Review

Multiple Choice

1. The functions of the digestive system include all except
   a. breakdown of food.
   b. absorption of nutrients.
   c. elimination of wastes.
   d. transportation of nutrients.

2. Peristalsis, chewing, and swallowing are part of
   a. mechanical digestion.
   b. chemical digestion.
   c. absorption.
   d. assimilation.

3. Chemical digestion involves
   a. the effects of bile, stomach acid, and enzymes on changing digested food into absorbable nutrient molecules.
   b. chewing.
   c. mastication.
   d. peristalsis.

4. Proteins become __________ when they have been chemically digested.
   a. glucose
   b. amino acids
   c. glycerol
   d. fatty acids

5. The end product, or absorbable nutrient, of carbohydrate digestion is
   a. glucose.
   b. amino acid.
   c. glycerol.
   d. fatty acid.

6. An adult has ___________ secondary teeth.
   a. 18
   b. 24
   c. 32
   d. 38

7. The parotid, submandibular, and sublingual glands produce
   a. bile.
   b. insulin.
   c. hydrochloric acid.
   d. saliva.

8. The ___________ is a muscular organ that lies on the left side of the upper quadrant of the abdominal cavity.
   a. esophagus
   b. stomach
   c. liver
   d. gall bladder

9. The sections of the small intestine include duodenum and
   a. jejunum and pylorus.
   b. ileum and colon.
   c. jejunum and ileum.
   d. cecum and jejunum.

10. Which organ of the alimentary canal is a muscular tube that is approximately 5 feet long?
    a. anus
    b. colon
    c. cecum
    d. jejunum

11. Functions of the liver include all except
    a. production of bile.
    b. conversion of glucose.
    c. neutralization of chemicals.
    d. storage of bile.

12. Which organ of the digestive system is an exocrine and endocrine gland?
    a. stomach
    b. gall bladder
    c. pancreas
    d. liver

13. Contribution factors to peptic ulcer formation include all except
    a. chronic stress.
    b. excessive histamine release.
    c. chronic gastritis.
    d. spicy foods.

14. The surgical procedure that produces a new opening for the removal of solid waste products from the colon is a
    a. colostomy.
    b. coloma.
    c. colectomy.
    d. cecumectomy.

15. A surgical procedure to create a new opening for removal of fecal waste products from the last part of the small intestine is called
    a. cecostomy.
    b. ileostomy.
    c. colostomy.
    d. jejunostomy.

Identification Exercise

Label the figure below:

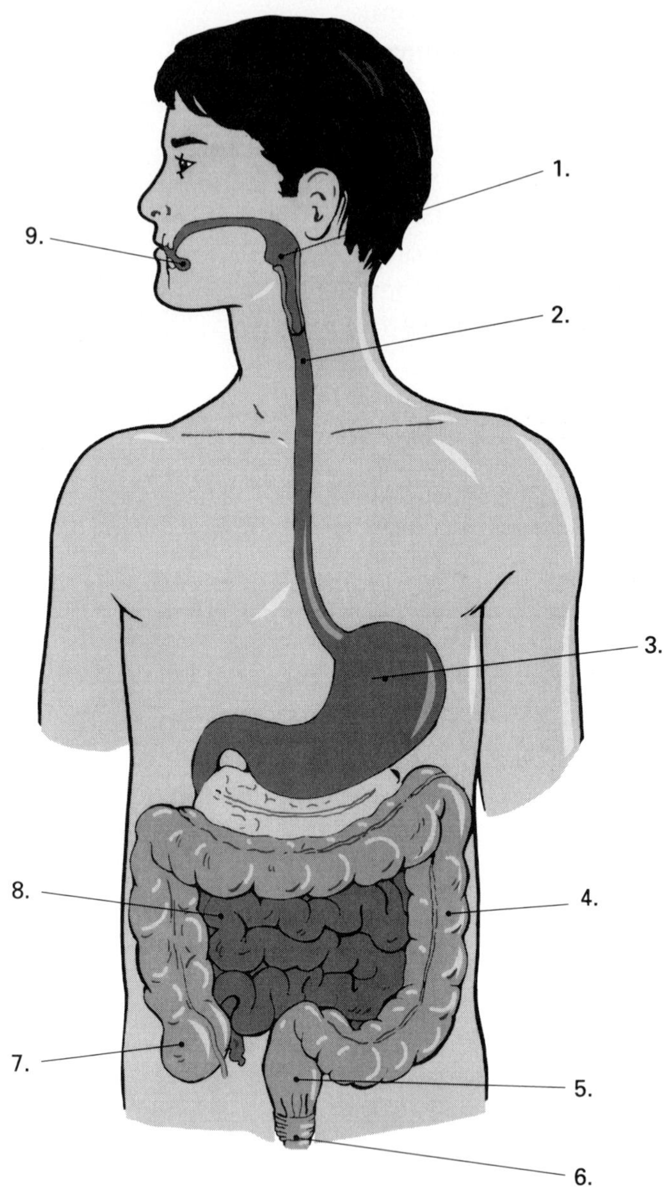

1. ___________________________   6. ___________________________

2. ___________________________   7. ___________________________

3. ___________________________   8. ___________________________

4. ___________________________   9. ___________________________

5. ___________________________

Vocabulary Activity

The following word search puzzle contains terms that are found in this chapter. Use the word list below to locate the hidden words in the grid.

```
M J E D O B R Z N P Z J K W P M C P R S
E E D N U J O I N A Q S P S W G E S P O
P J L F C O L O N N V U B Q I F V P A Q
S U T E R X D U E U T G W I O T D W U D
F N P A N C R E A S H J O U Q T V I E S
H U U K P A G Y N F J A G Q P U T E L K
V M J M O H I L E U M T R G S Z Z W B H
G P E R I T O N E U M P U B P J F J D F
M A S T I C A T I O N P G J E T E M X D
C L L M A N D I B L E L A W T L D Z F N
H A S L S B I N G U O R E D V U B K T S
R T Q P B D O X Y E Z P N P W Y P Q F I
W E Y T U L B L I V E R Z V O S N S F D
E L I M I N A T I O N H Y O I D N A A I
R Q K L W P N D V S J S M D S L C E R B
C T K Z L Y Q U D R M F E D Z C L D V D
W W B B U F P C P E R I S T A L S I S P
L D Q S W F H E P A R I N X C Z U Q M R
J S B Y L U X W P U W I T M G O Q A V H
K N E C D J V Y J A Z V F F K Q T Q T H
```

1. anus	12. mandible
2. colon	13. mastication
3. duodenum	14. melena
4. elimination	15. metabolism
5. enzymes	16. palate
6. gallbladder	17. pancreas
7. heparin	18. peristalsis
8. hyoid	19. peritoneum
9. ileum	20. rugae
10. jejunum	21. villi
11. liver	

Developing Vocabulary

Writing Practice

Beside each word below, write a complete sentence using the word. For each sentence, check for accuracy of content, spelling, and punctuation.

1. villi ____

    ____

    ____

2. anus ____

    ____

    ____

3. gallbladder ____

    ____

    ____

4. melena ____

    ____

    ____

5. liver ____

    ____

    ____

6. peritoneum ____

    ____

    ____

7. pancreas ____

    ____

    ____

8. duodenum ____

    ____

    ____

True or False

If the definition on the right corresponds to the word on the left, then check True, if the word and definition do not correspond, check False.

TRUE	FALSE	WORD
____	____	1. **Liver:** accessory organ vital to the process of digestion and absorption of nutrients
____	____	2. **Enzymes:** the contraction of the smooth muscle tissue that moves food along the intestines
____	____	3. **Hyoid:** process by which the teeth tear, grind, and chew food
____	____	4. **Peritoneum:** last part of the small intestine
____	____	5. **Heparin:** an exocrine and endocrine gland that produces two hormones and digestive enzymes

Spell Correctly

In each of the sets of words below, one word is spelled correctly. Circle the correctly spelled word.

1. a. poristalsis   c. peristalsis
    b. peirstalsis   d. peristaltis

2. a. masticatoin   c. masticatio
    b. masticatiinn   d. masticasion

3. a. jejunum   c. jnjunum
    b. jejunam   d. jejnnum

4. a. iluem   c. ileim
    b. ileam   d. ileum

5. a. metabolism   c. metobolism
    b. mteabolism   d. metabolasm

Practice Scenario(s)

After reading this chapter in the text, read the following scenario(s) and answer the questions following each of them.

Situation 1

Mr. Schnyder tells you that he has had a severe pain on his right side for about three hours. Two hours ago, his wife gave him an enema because she thought he was constipated. The pain intensified after the enema. When the doctor comes into the room to obtain a history and physical, Mr. Schnyder does not tell him about the enema.

1. Should you tell the doctor about the enema?

____

____

____

2. The physician asks Mr. Schnyder to locate the pain, and he points to his left side. What is unusual about the difference in the patient's location of the pain?

____

____

____

3. Is it important to tell the doctor, and why?

____

____

____

Situation 2

Ms. Jones is a 48-year-old mother of three who is a patient familiar to you. She has a diagnosis of ulcerative colitis. She has been admitted to your medical unit several times over the past three years. In report, the nurse said, "She was admitted yesterday with a flare-up of the symptoms, and she is dehydrated."

1. What does the diagnosis mean to you?

____

____

____

2. What is the "flare-up" of symptoms to which the nurse is referring?

____

____

____

3. Why would she be dehydrated?

____

____

____

Situation 3

Ms. Jones has had a colostomy. Ms. Jones becomes angry when you ask her to explain why she is crying and what she means about being "disfigured." You did not mean any harm; you just wanted to clarify what she was feeling.

1. Do you have any resources of people who can help Ms. Jones and you deal with your feelings?

____

____

____

Situation 4

Mrs. Avalon is a 38-year-old woman with insulin-dependent DM (IDDM). She was admitted to the ER at 2:00 A.M. in an unconscious state with a reaction.

1. What is her diagnosis, and why was she brought to the ER?

____

____

____

Situation 5

The RN asks you to obtain a blood glucose on Mrs. Avalon.

1. Why?

____

____

____

2. How can you do this?

____

____

____

Situation 6

Mr. Aramingo is a 40-year-old man who was admitted to your unit yesterday. In report, the nurse tells you that he has a GI bleed and must be closely monitored for bleeding. You are instructed to heme-test all stool and any emesis.

1. What is a hemetest?

____

____

____

2. What is emesis?

____

____

____

Situation 7

While you are caring for Mr. Aramingo, he has an episode of vomiting. You look at the contents of the basin and find emesis that looks like wet coffee grinds. You cannot imagine what happened because the patient has been NPO since admission.

1. What should you do?

____

____

____

Situation 8

When you return to Mr. Aramingo, you find that the skin is moist and cool. He is lethargic and tells you he needs the bedpan. You give him the bedpan, and his stool is very dark and almost looks like tar.

1. What do you do?

____

____

____

Situation 9

Mrs. Jenge is a 30-year-old woman whom you meet, for the first time, after the evening shift report. You find that Mrs. Jenge is a Caucasian woman whose skin is very yellow.

1. What do you think is the cause of this yellow skin condition?

____

____

____

Situation 10

The nurse tells you that Mrs. Jenge has hepatitis type A and that she was admitted because of dehydration.

1. What is hepatitis A, and how could she have acquired this condition?

____

____

____

Situation 11

You remember that you cared for another patient with hepatitis. This man had skin discoloration like Mrs. Jenge, but you were told that he had HBV.

1. What was the condition, and what was the difference about his hepatitis?

____

____

____

The Urinary System

Chapter Review

Multiple Choice

1. The functions of the urinary system include all of the following except
   a. production and elimination of urine.
   b. elimination of excess salts and water.
   c. maintenance of acid/base balance.
   d. elimination of fatty acids and protein.

2. The kidneys are located in the
   a. retroperitoneal space.
   b. retrothoracic space.
   c. anterioabdominal cavity.
   d. anteriopelvic cavity.

3. Which organ produces urine?
   a. bladder
   b. kidney
   c. ureter
   d. urethra

4. The microscopic working units of the kidneys are called
   a. medullas.
   b. nephrons.
   c. capsules.
   d. neurons.

5. The sections of a nephron include all except
   a. glomerulus.
   b. Bowman's capsule.
   c. renal tubules.
   d. pyramids.

6. The water retaining hormone is
   a. aldosterone.
   b. diuretic hormone.
   c. antidiuretic hormone.
   d. albuterol.

7. What should NOT be found in normal urine?
   a. water
   c. protein
   b. sodium
   d. potassium

8. A test that measures the concentration of water in urine is
   a. specific gravity.
   b. pH concentration.
   c. urine culture.
   d. C&S.

9. The structures that drain urine from the renal pelvis to the bladder are
   a. nephrons.
   c. urethras.
   b. hilums.
   d. ureters.

10. Which organ is located in the pelvic cavity anterior to the rectum?
    a. bladder
    c. kidney
    b. renal pelvis
    d. urethra

11. Which microorganism is often the cause of cystitis?
    a. streptococcus
    c. E. Coli
    b. staphylococcus
    d. clostridium

12. Infection, immobility, and dehydration are usual causes of
    a. pyelonephritis.
    b. cystitis.
    c. renal failure.
    d. renal calculi.

13. Treatments for renal failure include all but
    a. hemodialysis.
    b. peritoneal dialysis.
    c. gamma globulin.
    d. increased fluids.

14. The female urethra measures approximately __________ inches.
    a. 4–5
    c. 6–8
    b. 2–3
    d. 5–7

15. The tuft of capillaries that acts as a filter in the nephron is the
    a. renal tubule.
    b. glomerulus.
    c. Bowman's capsule.
    d. renal arteriole.

Identification Exercise

Label the figure below:

1. _________________________   8. _________________________

2. _________________________   9. _________________________

3. _________________________   10. ________________________

4. _________________________   11. ________________________

5. _________________________   12. ________________________

6. _________________________   13. ________________________

7. _________________________   14. ________________________

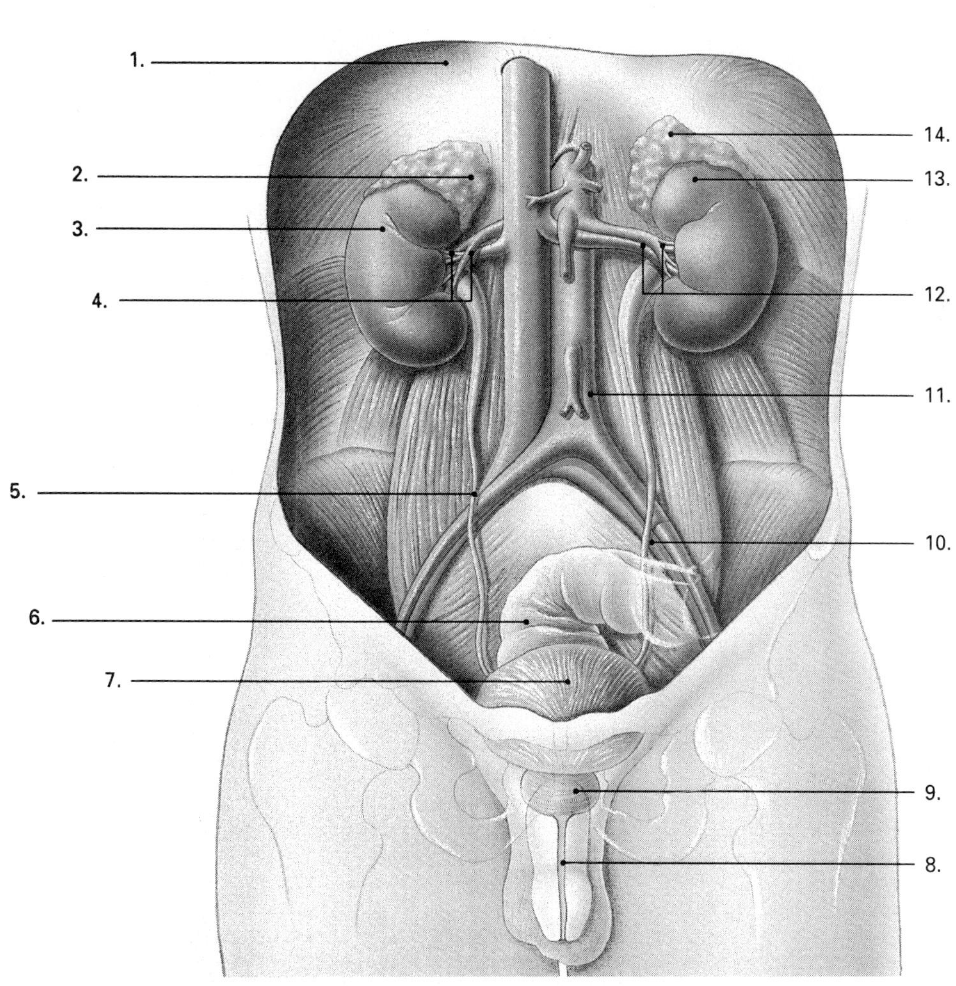

Vocabulary Activity

The following crossword puzzle contains terms that are found in this chapter. Use the clues below to complete the puzzle.

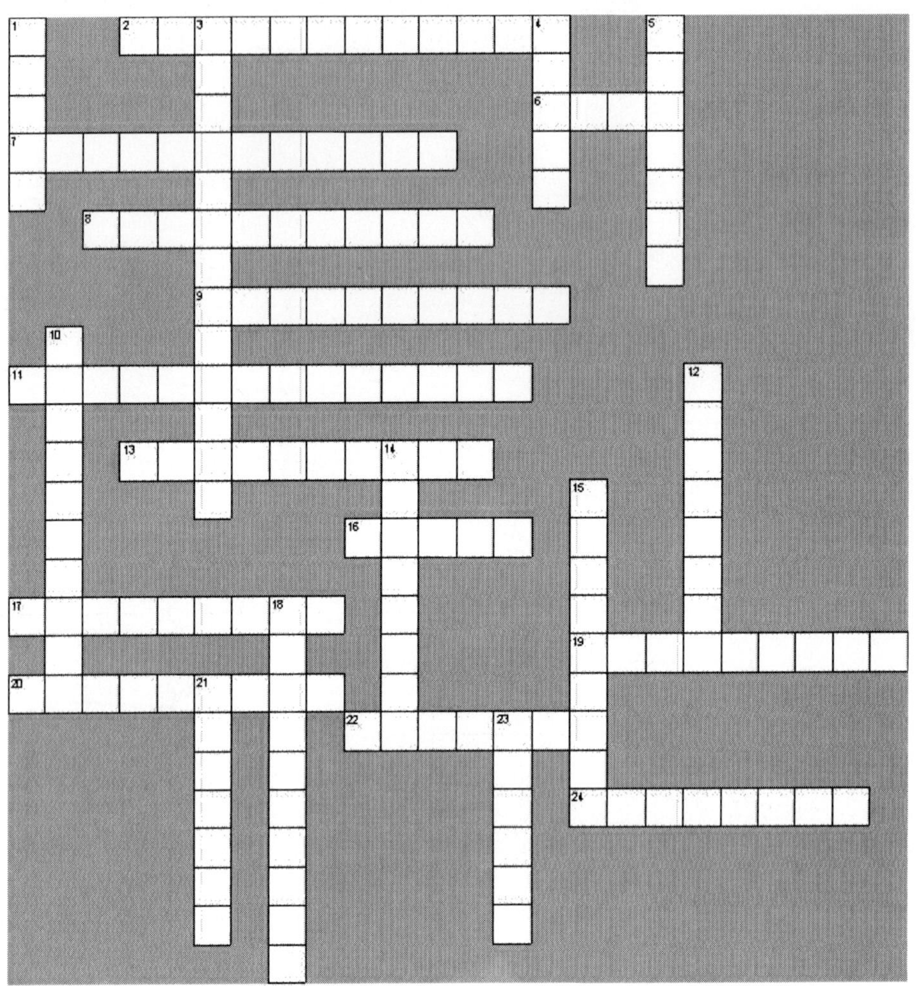

ACROSS

2. lifesaving procedure of artificially purifying the blood when kidneys fail
6. byproduct of protein metabolism
7. surgical creation of a new opening for urine excretion from the body
8. salt-retaining hormone that regulates urine production
9. cluster of capillaries in the nephron
11. inflammation of the kidneys and renal pelvis
13. removal of the bladder
16. depression in the kidney where the blood vessels enter and exit
17. important electrolyte necessary in urine production
19. bloodstream infection due to the buildup of waste products when the kidneys fail
20. blood in the urine
22. stones formed in the kidneys
24. microscopic working units of the kidney

DOWN

1. thick fluid secreted by mucous membranes
3. small living thing invisible to the naked eye
4. artificial connection of an artery and vein used in hemodialysis
5. muscular reservoir for urine storage before excretion from the body
10. instrument used to visually examine the bladder
12. inflammation of the bladder
14. very small amount of urine formation
15. passage of fluid from an area of greater concentration to lesser concentration
18. laboratory analysis of urine to detect abnormalities in pH, color, or constituents
21. tubular passageway from the bladder for urine excretion from the body
23. long, narrow tubular passageway extending from the kidneys to the bladder

Developing Vocabulary

Writing Practice

Beside each word below, write a complete sentence using the word. For each sentence, check for accuracy of content, spelling, and punctuation.

1. urosepsis _______________________________________

____

____

2. hilum_______________________________________

____

____

3. potassium _______________________________________

____

____

4. cystectomy _______________________________________

____

____

5. diffusion _______________________________________

____

____

6. microorganism_______________________________________

____

____

7. urea _______________________________________

____

____

8. urinalysis _______________________________________

____

____

True or False

If the definition on the right corresponds to the word on the left, then check True, if the word and definition do not correspond, check False.

TRUE   FALSE   WORD

____   ____   1. **Ureterostomy:** surgical creation of a new opening for urine excretion from the body

____   ____   2. **Hematuria:** tubular passageway from the bladder for urine excretion

____   ____   3. **Shunt:** an artificial connection of an artery and vein used in hemodialysis

___   ___   4. **Mucus:** a thick fluid secreted by mucous membranes

____   ____   5. **Cystoscope:** Instrument used to visually examine the bladder

Spell Correctly

In each of the sets of words below, one word is spelled correctly. Circle the correctly spelled word.

1.   a. aldosetrone   c. aldasterone
      b. aldusterone   d. aldosterone

2.   a. guomerulus   c. glemerulus
      b. glomerolus   d. glomerulus

3.   a. oleguria   c. oligeria
      b. oliuuria   d. oliguria

4.   a. pyelonephrisis   c. pyelonaphritis
      b. pyelonephritis   d. pyelonophritis

5.   a. cystctis   c. cyititis
      b. cyssitis   d. cystitis

Practice Scenario(s)

After reading this chapter in the text, read the following scenario(s) and answer the questions following each of them.

Situation 1

Mrs. Dell's diagnosis was **urosepsis** resulting from pyelonephritis and cystitis. She was treated with IV antibiotics and within three days her WBC count of 18.9 was reduced to 10.7. Her temperature was normal.

1. What does her diagnosis indicate about the organs that were infected?

____

____

____

2. What is the significance of the WBC changes?

____

____

____

Situation 2

Mr. Isreal is a patient on the oncology unit. He was admitted for surgical removal of his urinary bladder and prostate gland because of malignant tumors. Mr. Isreal had a cystectomy with prostatectomy.

1. How will Mr. Isreal excrete his urine?

____

____

____

2. What must you consider in your observation and care of Mr. Isreal concerning his ureterostomy?

____

____

____

Situation 3

Ms. Kim is a patient on the rehab unit. She has an indwelling urinary catheter. The nurse tells you that Ms. Kim has cystitis.

1. Where is the catheter?

____

____

____

2. What is cystitis?

____

____

____

3. Why might Ms. Kim have cystitis?

____

____

____

Situation 4

You are working on a pediatric rehabilitation unit in an LTC. You are assigned to John Kniezweski, an 8-year-old boy who has paraplegia. He has an indwelling Foley catheter, and he had a colostomy three months ago. At 8:00 A.M. John rings his call bell to tell you that his "tummy" hurts. When you check his ostomy appliance you see that it is full of liquid stool, so you empty it. At 9:00 A.M., you return to his room, and he complains of cramps in his tummy; once again, you find the colostomy appliance is full of liquid stool. John looks sad and tells you he did not eat yesterday, and he doesn't want to eat today. He refuses any liquids and just wants to stay in his room. At 3:00 P.M., you empty his urinary drainage bag and it has only 100 cc of urine. His colostomy appliance is full of liquid stool.

1. What do you do with this information?

____

____

____

2. What do you think is the connection between a small amount of urine and a large amount of liquid stool (diarrhea)?

____

____

____

C h a p t e r   1 5

The Reproductive System

Chapter Review

Multiple Choice

1. The function of the scrotum is to
   a. protect the penis.
   b. house the testes.
   c. prevent infection.
   d. produce testosterone.

2. The surgical procedure that removes the foreskin of the penis is a
   a. vasectomy.
   b. circumcision.
   c. prepuce.
   d. testectomy.

3. Which structure produces spermatozoa?
   a. ductus deferens
   b. epididymis
   c. seminiferous tubules
   d. vas deferens

4. Which of the following glands does NOT produce seminal fluid?
   a. prostate
   b. bulbourethral
   c. seminal vesicles
   d. Bartholin's

5. The normal twenty-third (23rd) pair of chromosomes in a male is indicated as
   a. XX.
   b. YY.
   c. XY.
   d. YYX.

6. The most common type of cancer in American males over the age of 50 is
   a. testicular.
   b. prostate.
   c. bladder.
   d. scrotal.

7. Which STD presents with a chancre or sore on the genitals or lips and may also cause rash, fever, and swollen lymph nodes?
   a. herpes
   b. chlamydia
   c. syphilis
   d. gonorrhea

8. The external genitalia of a female are collectively referred to as
   a. labia majora.
   b. vagina.
   c. clitoris.
   d. vulva.

9. The female gonad is the
   a. vagina.
   b. ovary.
   c. ovum.
   d. fallopian tubes.

10. What happens when a Graafian follicle ruptures and an ovum is released?
    a. menstruation
    b. pregnancy
    c. menarche
    d. ovulation

11. The organ responsible for menstruation, implantation of the fertilized egg, and labor is the
    a. ovary.
    b. uterus.
    c. fallopian tube.
    d. vagina.

12. Which are the organs of copulation?
    a. testes and ovaries
    b. uterus and epididymis
    c. vagina and penis
    d. penis and clitoris

13. Which hormone is responsible for the production and let-down of milk in the female breasts?
    a. oxytocin
    b. pitocin
    c. estrogen
    d. progesterone

14. A test to detect the presence of abnormal cells of the cervix is the
    a. mammogram.
    b. Pap test.
    c. cervical self-exam.
    d. hysterosalpingogram.

15. When should breast self-exams be performed by a woman?
    a. when a lump is suspected
    b. during her menses
    c. after her menstrual period has ended
    d. daily after a shower

Vocabulary Activity

The following word search puzzle contains terms that are found in this chapter. Use the word list below to locate the hidden words in the grid.

```
S T Q M T R U G G Y Q B D C I C C P T Y
C A S J E N D O M E T R I U M O L I E S
R E L D O B F R M T F E T U S I I M D Y
O P R P P L A C E N T A X H E B T N R E
T V Z V I A N H V I D S Z W Y E O D V F
U F U X I N V I I N S T N B I M R Q O I
M J I L B X G D V P S S B H H A I H O M
S G O N A D A E P I D I D Y M I S D N B
N M J Z E T E C C O P U L A T I O N W R
F K T O J W I T Z T K M Q I W E X M A I
Q B I H R O K O M Y O M E T R I U M D A
H C S W I T C M N O G M E N O P A U S E
B G J D S E G Y W W V O Y Z A L S O O M
L E N W O S S V U L V A T S F R Z F E A
C Y X H R Z B E H F M P R E P U C E W Q
P C X L T K D J L E V N H Y M E N H M J
U M U G W H K D Q K V S M B U T R D E X
D P B N H H V B Z R M L M U A S L M U W
M N F B O A B H V V U L O I P V B E Q S
W V D T V R M Z I M I R E V J I N O V U
```

1. breasts	13. menopause
2. cervix	14. myometrium
3. clitoris	15. orchidectomy
4. copulation	16. ovary
5. endometrium	17. ovulation
6. epididymis	18. placenta
7. fetus	19. prepuce
8. fimbriae	20. salginpectomy
9. fundus	21. scrotum
10. gonad	22. sperm
11. hymen	23. vulva
12. menarche	24. zygote

Developing Vocabulary

Writing Practice

Beside each word below, write a complete sentence using the word. For each sentence, check for accuracy of content, spelling, and punctuation.

1. zygote ____

____

____

2. breasts ____

____

____

3. salginpectomy ____________________________________

____

____

4. menopause ____

____

____

5. sperm ____

____

____

6. orchidectomy ______________________________________

____

____

7. fetus ____

____

____

8. endometrium ______________________________________

____

____

True or False

If the definition on the right corresponds to the word on the left, then check True, if the word and definition do not correspond, check False.

TRUE	FALSE	WORD
____	____	1. **Prepuce:** the inner layer of the uterus
____	____	2. **Endometrium:** mammary glands that produce and release milk to nourish an infant
____	____	3. **Fundus:** the bulging upper part of the uterus
____	____	4. **Hymen:** unborn human developing in the uterus after the eighth week of pregnancy
____	____	5. **Cervix:** the neck of the uterus at the inferior end, which opens to the vagina

Spell Correctly

In each of the sets of words below, one word is spelled correctly. Circle the correctly spelled word.

1.   a. epadidymis   c. epudidymis
         b. eiididymis   d. epididymis

2.   a. manarche   c. menarche
         b. menerche   d. minarche

3.   a. plaeentra   c. placenta
         b. plecenta   d. plicenta

4.   a. myometiium   c. myometruim
         b. myometrium   d. myemetrium

5.   a. copulatian   c. copulation
         b. copulition   d. copolation

Practice Scenario(s)

After reading this chapter in the text, read the following scenario(s) and answer the questions following each of them.

Situation 1

Mr. Clemens is a 70-year-old man who is experiencing both difficulty starting a stream of urine and pain upon urination. His diagnosis is BPH. He is scheduled for surgery for a TURP. You are the clinical care associate (CCA) working in the recovery room.

On Mr. Clemens's third post-op day, you are expected to observe and measure the contents of the urinary drainage bag. When you make morning rounds, you find that there is no drainage in the bag. The night shift I & O (intake and output) accounts for 200 cc of output at 6 A.M. It is now 8 A.M.

1. What do you expect will be the status of this patient post-op?

   ____

   ____

   ____

2. What action will you take regarding no drainage in the urinary drainage bag?

   ____

   ____

   ____

Situation 2

You are the CCA working on the OB-GYN unit. A 22-year-old female is admitted to your unit with severe abdominal pain and fever. Her last menstrual period (LMP) was 8 weeks ago. The initial diagnosis is rule out (r\o) ectopic pregnancy. This 22-year-old is not pregnant. She is diagnosed with PID.

1. Why would the diagnosis of ectopic pregnancy be suspected?

   ____

   ____

   ____

2. What are the causes and symptoms of PID?

____

____

____

Situation 3

Mrs. Shore is a 45-year-old mother of four children. She arrives in the emergency room (ER) with complaints of (c\o) a "very heavy period." She tells you that she has used seven pads in the past 2 hours. The nurse directs you to lower the head of the bed, to keep Mrs. Shore in bed, and to monitor her VS every 15 minutes. She increases the drip rate of the IV fluids. The ultrasound reveals a large growth in the uterus, and a CT scan is ordered. Mrs. Shore continues to saturate the perineal pads at the rate of one pad every 30 minutes. Her pulse is thready, and her BP is not audible. She is not responsive when you try to check her perineal pad.

1. What is the term for excessive menstrual flow?

____

____

____

2. What do you do regarding the fact that Mrs. Jenkins is not responsive when you try to check her perineal pad?

____

____

____

3. How can you measure the patient's BP if you cannot hear it with the stethoscope?

____

____

____

Situation 4

Mrs. Jenkins is a 38-year old who has a history of fibrocystic breast disease. She routinely performs breast self-exams. This month, she notes a non-tender lump in the RUQ of her right breast. In addition, she has lost 10 pounds in the past three months, which she attributed to the stress of her new job. Her last gynecological exam was six months ago. When Mrs. Jenkins has her gyn exam, the physician confirms Mrs. Jenkins' suspicions. She is scheduled for hospitalization. The surgical consult form says: "Breast Bx possible R mastectomy." Mrs. Jenkins asks you, the CCA, why the physician wrote this. The pathologist confirms the presence of malignant cells in Mrs. Jenkins's frozen section.

1. What action should Mrs. Jenkins have taken when she discovered the non-tender lump in her right breast?

   ____

   ____

   ____

2. When is the best time to perform breast self-exams?

   ____

   ____

   ____

3. When Mrs. Jenkins asks you why the physician write: "Breast Bx possible R mastectomy," what do you tell her?

   ____

   ____

   ____

4. What is your next action?

   ____

   ____

   ____

5. What does the term *frozen section* mean?

   ____

   ____

   ____

The Endocrine System

Chapter Reivew

Multiple Choice

1. Endocrine glands differ from exocrine glands because they
   a. bypass the bloodstream.
   b. employ vessels.
   c. utilize enzymes.
   d. lack ducts.

2. Which structure of the brain controls the functions of the pituitary gland?
   a. thalmus
   b. hypopituitary
   c. hypothalmus
   d. cerebrum

3. Which hormone of the anterior pituitary stimulates the growth and secretion of the adrenal cortex?
   a. TSH
   b. FSH
   c. ACTH
   d. LH

4. Dwarfism is caused by hyposecretion of
   a. GH.
   b. ACTH.
   c. LH.
   d. TSH.

5. The hormone secreted excessively in acute stress situations is
   a. aldosterone.
   b. epinephrine.
   c. glucagon.
   d. insulin.

6. The water-retaining hormone is
   a. diuretic hormone.
   b. aldosterone.
   c. antidiuretic hormone.
   d. cortisone.

7. Which gland produces hormones that accelerate cellular metabolism?
   a. adrenal
   b. thyroid
   c. pituitary
   d. parathyroid

8. Which hormone regulates blood calcium levels?
   a. calcitonin
   b. epinephrine
   c. thyroxin
   d. insulin

9. Epinephrine and norepinephrine are produced and secreted by which gland?
   a. adrenal cortex
   b. posterior pituitary
   c. adrenal medulla
   d. anterior pituitary

10. Which hormone works to decrease the amount of glucose in circulating in the blood?
    a. androgen
    b. glucocorticoids
    c. insulin
    d. glucagon

11. Estrogen does not affect
    a. breast development.
    b. placenta formation.
    c. calcium storage.
    d. sex drive.

12. Which structure produces progesterone?
    a. seminepherous tubules
    b. graafin follicle
    c. corpus luteum
    d. mammary gland

13. Cushing's syndrome is caused by all but the following.
    a. tumor of the adrenal cortex
    b. prolonged use of steroids
    c. excessive secretion of ACTH
    d. burnout of the adrenal medulla

14. One of the treatments for IDDM is
    a. oral hypoglycemics.
    b. low fat diet.
    c. insulin injections.
    d. IV glucagon.

15. Which of the following is caused by hyposecretion of ADH?
    a. diabetes insipidus
    b. exophthalmic goiter
    c. Addison's disease
    d. Grave's disease

Vocabulary Activity

The following crossword puzzle contains terms that are found in this chapter. Use the clues below to complete the puzzle.

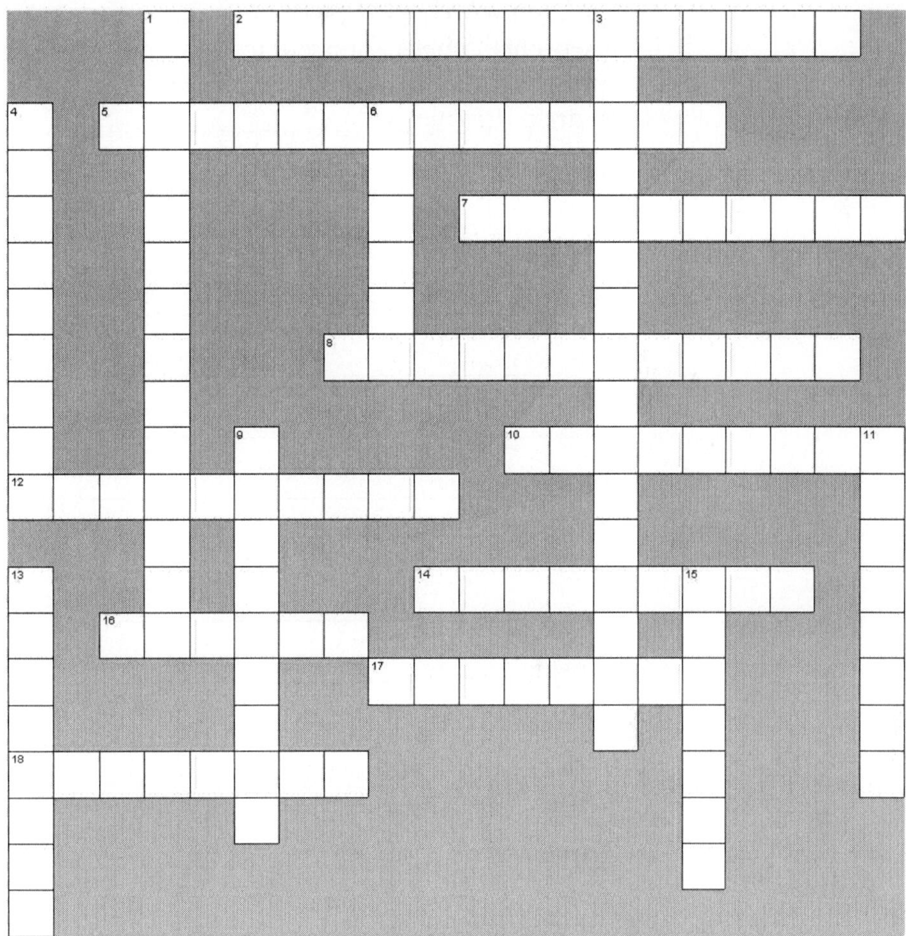

ACROSS

2. corticosteroid hormone
5. local, tissue hormones
7. abnormal enlargement of the extremities
8. female hormone necessary for maintaining pregnancy
10. hormone produced by the thyroid gland
12. pertaining to the area above the kidneys
14. result of an excess production of growth hormone causing excess growth greater than seven feet
16. hyperactivity of the muscles
17. chemical messengers of the body
18. caused by hyposecretion of growth hormone, resulting in short stature

DOWN

1. adrenal cortex hormone influencing CHO, K, and Na metabolism
3. T4, thyroid hormone
4. male sex hormones
6. enlargement of the thyroid gland
9. anterior pituitary hormone that promotes lactation
11. female hormone that helps maintain feminine characteristics
13. disease that results from hypofunction of the thyroid gland
15. hormone that works to decrease the mount of circulating glucose

Developing Vocabulary

Writing Practice

Beside each word below, write a complete sentence using the word. For each sentence, check for accuracy of content, spelling, and punctuation.

1. hydrocortisone

2. ductless

3. thyroxine

4. prostaglandins

5. progesterone

6. suprarenal

7. hormones

8. tetany

True or False

If the definition on the right corresponds to the word on the left, then check True, if the word and definition do not correspond, check False.

TRUE	FALSE	WORD
____	____	1. **Androgens:** male sex hormones
____	____	1. **Goiter:** hormone that works to decrease the amount of circulating glucose
____	____	1. **Thyroxine:** hormone produced by the thyroid gland
____	____	1. **Myxedema:** chemical messengers of the body
____	____	1. **Dwarfism:** anterior pituitary hormone that promotes lactation

Spell Correctly

In each of the sets of words below, one word is spelled correctly. Circle the correctly spelled word.

1.
   a. certicosterone
   b. corticostreone
   c. corticosteorne
   d. corticosterone

2.
   a. prolactin
   b. prelactin
   c. prolictin
   d. prolectin

3.
   a. acromegily
   b. acromegaly
   c. acromeguly
   d. acromogaly

4.
   a. epanephrine
   b. epinephrine
   c. epenephrine
   d. eprnephrine

5.
   a. triiotothyronine
   b. triiodothyrenine
   c. triiodothyronine
   d. triiodothyronene

Practice Scenario(s)

After reading this chapter in the text, read the following scenario(s) and answer the questions following each of them.

Situation 1

Mrs. Bickel is a 63-year-old woman with diabetes mellitus. She has been on insulin for two years. Mrs. Bickel self-administers 40 u of NPH q.d. Mrs. Bickel is admitted to the medical unit. She c/o "not feeling right." Her physician's note reads: pt. has been experiencing polyuria, polydipsia, and polyphagia. What do the terms polyuria, polydipsia, and polyphagia. mean to you? Her physician's admission note also indicates that she has a small ulceration on her R big toe. Her FBS today was 310. 5. The Kardex states:"Never cut this patient's toe nails." Her physician increased her insulin dose to 55 units of NPH with a sliding scale for regular insulin based on the q. 6 hour blood glucose monitoring. In the afternoon you enter Mrs. Bickel's room and find her unresponsive. Her skin feels hot and dry, and her respirations are slow and deep. The next morning before breakfast, Mrs. Bickel rings the call bell. You enter her room and find her sweating, her hands are shaking, and she says, "I am starving. The nurse gave me my insulin and I need to eat."

1. What type of Diabetes does she have?

   ____

   ____

   ____

2. You know that Mrs. Bickel self-administers 40 u of NPH q.d. What does this mean?

   ____

   ____

   ____

3. What do the terms polyuria, polydipsia, and polyphagia mean to you?

   ____

   ____

   ____

4. She has a small ulceration on her R big toe. Her FBS today was 310. What does this mean to you?

____

____

____

5. Why does the Kardex state that you should never cut this patient's toe nails?

____

____

____

6. What does it mean to you that her physician increased her insulin dose to 55 units of NPH with a sliding scale for regular insulin based on the q. 6 hour blood glucose monitoring?

____

____

____

7. When you find Mrs. Bickel's unresponsive in the afternoon, with skin that feels hot and dry and respirations that are slow and deep, what do you do?

____

____

____

8. What could have happened to Mrs. Bickel?

____

____

____

9. Why do you think that Mrs. Bickel is so hungry, sweaty, and shaky when you enter her room the next morning before breakfast?

____

____

____

10. What will you do?

____

____

____

Situation 2

Ms. March is a 56 year old woman who was admitted from the ER to the MICU because of delirium, bradycardia and hypotonic muscle and nervous responses. You are assigned to Ms. March, and the nurse asks you to draw an ionized calcium. She reminds you to wrap the vaccutainer tube for blood sample in aluminum foil to protect it from exposure to light.

1. Why would you be directed to draw an ionized calcium?

____

____

____

2. What could have caused an increased blood calcium and these symptoms?

____

____

____

A Nursing-Process Approach to Care Delivery

Chapter Review

Multiple Choice

1. Which is not a characteristic of objective data?
   a. measurable
   b. factual
   c. descriptive
   d. subjective

2. Gathering equipment is which step in the nursing process?
   a. assess
   b. plan
   c. implement
   d. evaluate

3. Which is NOT a specified factor in the RN's delegation of a task to the CCA?
   a. patient status
   b. task complexity
   c. possible harm
   d. outcome predictability

4. Acting in the best interest of the patient to produce greater good than harm represents
   a. autonomy.
   b. beneficence.
   c. justice.
   d. non-maleficence.

5. Collaboration, communication, contribution, cooperation, and commitment are the foundation of
   a. ethics.
   b. licensure.
   c. teamwork.
   d. continuity.

6. Forms of verbal communication include all of the following except
   a. body gestures.
   b. spoken words.
   c. phone calls.
   d. written language.

7. Lack of knowledge and receptive aphasia are examples of
   ___________ barriers to communication.
   a. physical
   b. mental
   c. emotional
   d. cultural

8. Referring to a geriatric client as "Granny" could violate which
   patient right?
   a. confidentiality
   b. consent
   c. privacy
   d. respect

9. Discussing a patient's diagnosis with a co-worker publicly
   would violate which patient right?
   a. confidentiality
   b. identity
   c. respect
   d. consultation

10. Receiving report from the RN falls under which step of the
    nursing process?
    a. assessing
    b. planning
    c. implementing
    d. evaluating

11. A factor that does NOT shape the scope of practice for an LPN is
    a. state law.
    b. facility policy.
    c. job description.
    d. registry code.

12. CCA documentation about the patient's skin after a bed bath
    denotes
    a. assessing.
    b. planning.
    c. implementing.
    d. evaluating.

13. Considering patient's values demonstrates which ethical principle?
    a. beneficence   c. justice
    b. autonomy   d. non-maleficence

Vocabulary Activity

The following crossword puzzle contains terms that are found in this chapter. Use the clues below to complete the puzzle.

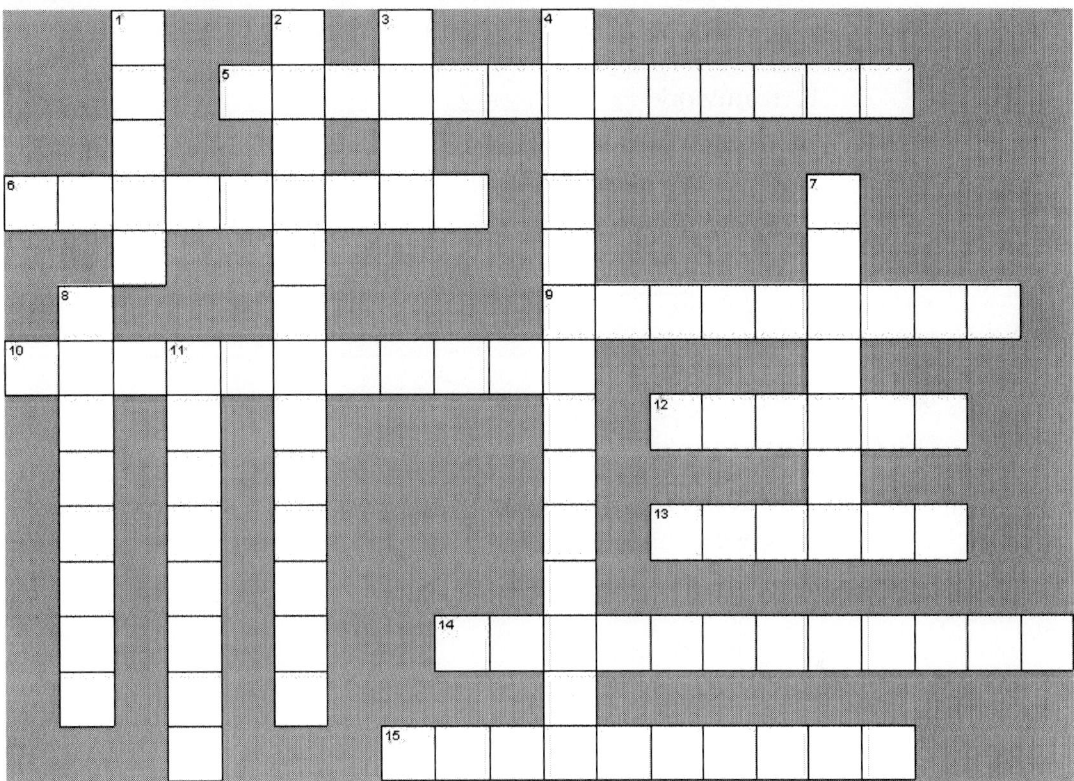

ACROSS

5. to combine efforts that independently are not as effective as when jointly performed
6. carry out the plan
9. assumption that the person who holds a license is deemed
10. professional will act in the best interests of the patient
12. a moral code and standards of conduct that guide professional behavior
13. gathering data to understand the situation
14. to give a part or have a share in any act or effect
15. the act of appointing tasks to others

DOWN

1. range or extent of an action, observation, or inquiry
2. imparting information that has been received
3. organizing the care to be delivered
4. professionals do not act in a manner knowingly harmful to the patient
7. fairness achieved by the equal distribution of costs and benefits
8. working together to provide the best care to patients
11. determining the results based on instructions given and patient response

Developing Vocabulary

Writing Practice

Beside each word below, write a complete sentence using the word. For each sentence, check for accuracy of content, spelling, and punctuation.

1. teamwork ____

____

____

2. ethics____

____

____

3. collaboration ____

____

____

4. contribution____

____

____

5. communication ____

____

____

6. beneficence ____

____

____

7. delegation____

____

____

8. evaluate____

____

____

True or False

If the definition on the right corresponds to the word on the left, then check True, if the word and definition do not correspond, check False.

TRUE	FALSE	WORD
____	____	1. **Scope:** range or extent of an action, observation, or inquiry
____	____	2. **Plan:** professionals do not act in a manner knowingly harmful to the patient
____	____	3. **Ethics:** a moral code and standard of conduct that guides
____	____	4. **Justice:** fairness is achieved by the equal distribution of costs and benefits
____	____	5. **Contribution:** to combine efforts that independently are not as effective as when jointly performed

Spell Correctly

In each of the sets of words below, one word is spelled correctly. Circle the correctly spelled word.

1. a. evaluite   c. evaluete
    b. evaleate   d. evaluate

2. a. cillaboration   c. collabaration
    b. cellaboration   d. collaboration

3. a. bineficence   c. beneficence
    b. beneficince   d. benefiience

4. a. licensure   c. licinsure
    b. licenssre   d. licensere

5. a. non-maleficence   c. non-mulificence
    b. non-malificence   d. non-malificnnce

Practice Scenario(s)

After reading this chapter in the text, read the following scenario(s) and answer the questions following each of them.

Situation 1

Mr. Smith is an 80-year-old man who resides in your nursing home. He has lived there for five years, and you have been involved in his care for four years. Has has been diagnosed with diabetes mellitus, hypertension, and, recently, a kidney infection. He will need a Foley catheter and an IV to manage his condition.

Mr. Smith has always been able to perform some of his personal care and ADLs, with assistance. He ambulates with use of a walker, is alert, and is socially active with other residents. He likes to play checkers, and he reads the paper daily. He also discusses what he reads with you. Today, Monday, you are assigned to Mr. Smith after being off for the weekend. As you make your rounds, you expect to find him sitting in a chair, eating his breakfast, and reading his paper. When you enter the room, he is in bed, and he is waiting for you to assist him with his breakfast. He tells you, "I feel weak and do not have much of an appetite. I'll just have the juice and coffee." You notice that his urinary drainage bag contains a small amount of very dark, reddish brown urine. He complains of a backache, so you raise the head of his bed to a sitting position. He appears sleepy and is slow to respond to your questions.

After you assist him with drinking his juice and coffee, you receive a report from the nurse. She directs you to provide A.M. care and to get Mr. Smith ready to attend a recreational activity at 10:00. She tells you he has a Heplock in his left arm for the administration of intravenous antibiotics and a Foley for accurate urinary measurement. He has been placed on I&O and was given Tylenol for pain during the night. During the report, you relate to the nurse the objective data collected on your rounds to Mr. Smith. The nurse tells you to increase Mr. Smith's oral intake of fluids. You encourage Mr. Smith to drink more water.

No instructions were given regarding a modification or alteration in A.M. care. You find that in performing Mr. Smith's A.M. care he can barely assist you because he is so lethargic. He does not want to get out of bed, and he refuses to attend the recreational activity because he is too weak. He also "does not want to be seen by other residents with a Foley." He has taken abut 300 cubic centimeters (cc) of fluids by mouth (PO), and at 11:00 A.M. you decide to measure the contents of the drainage bag. The output is 50 cc.

At noon, you take vital signs again because of the q4° order. The resulsts are temperature 100°F, pulse 110, respirations 28, blood pressure 180/100. Blood glucose measured via a fingerstick is 233 (normal range is 84-126). You are surprised because he hasn't eaten anything.

During the bath you notice that his feet are swollen and, when you touch them, you leave fingermarks on his skin. His IV of 1,000 cc of Dextrose 5% and 1/2% normal saline solution has infused about 75% of the bag. His breathing is labored; it seems to take much effort for him to wash his face.

1. Who will be permitted to insert the Foley catheter?

   ____

   ____

   ____

2. Who will insert the IV? What are your responsibilities in maintaining Mr. Smith's IV?

   ____

   ____

   ____

3. What are your responsibilities in maintaining Mr. Smith's urinary catheter?

   ____

   ____

   ____

4. How will your observations and the nurse's assessment affect the way you plan to carry out your assignment?

   ____

   ____

   ____

5. Will you alter your usual appraach to Mr. Smith's A.M. care? For what reasons will you alter your plan?

____

____

____

6. What are the objective data (measurements and observations) about Mr. Smith's condition that you have gathered? Describe your reasons for reporting this data. Should this data be assessed by the nurse?

____

____

____

7. In your own words, describe what you contributed to the nurse's assessment. What changes were made in the nurse's plan of care? What tasks were you assigned to implement? What data did you provide to assist the nurse in evaluating Mr. Smith's response to the plan of care?

____

____

____

8. What data did you gather through your senses?

____

____

____

9. What data did you gather through measurement?

____

____

____

Elementary Nutrition

Chapter Review

Multiple Choice

1. The resting rate of one's metabolism when no voluntary work is being done is called
   a. basal.
   b. assimilative.
   c. catabolic.
   d. anabolic.

2. Carbohydrates are broken down into
   a. amino acids.
   b. simple sugars.
   c. saturated fats.
   d. soluble vitamins.

3. Fluids are lost in the form of all BUT
   a. urine.
   b. sweat.
   c. stool.
   d. irrigation.

4. Grains and cereals are examples of
   a. complete proteins.
   b. amino acids.
   c. simple carbohydrates.
   d. complex CHO.

5. Ten (10) grams of fat provide the body with __________ calories.
   a. 9
   b. 90
   c. 40
   d. 4

6. Which food essential rebuilds and repairs tissues?
   a. fiber
   b. carbohydrate
   c. fat
   d. protein

7. Vitamin B_{12} is needed for
   a. RBC formation.
   b. skin tone.
   c. kidney function.
   d. cellular repair.

8. Which of the following vitamins does the body store?
   a. A, D
   b. C, K
   c. B, C
   d. B, E

9. The recommended intake of vegetables is __________ servings daily.
   a. 2-4
   b. 2-3
   c. 3-5
   d. 6-11

10. Which vitamin is needed for blood clotting?
    a. K
    b. E
    c. C
    d. B

11. Calorie restricted diets are indicated for
    a. renal disease.
    b. bowel disorders.
    c. weight loss.
    d. cholesterol reduction.

12. Foods to be avoid when reducing dangerous blood lipids are
    a. egg yolks and organ meats.
    b. bullion and salt.
    c. fish and beans.
    d. canned foods and prepacked items.

13. Foods such as broth, apple juice, ginger ale, and gelatin would be served to a patient on a __________ diet.
    a. low protein
    b. clear liquid
    c. low sodium
    d. full liquid

14. If a patient can digest food but cannot swallow, nutrition would be provided by a __________ tube.
    a. gastrostomy
    b. intravenous
    c. nasoesophageal
    d. ileostomy

15. Which characteristic of hyperalimentation is NOT true?
    a. provides calorie maintenance
    b. prescribed for malabsorption syndrome
    c. administered through peripheral veins
    d. supplies fluids and electrolytes

Identification Exercise

Label the figure below:

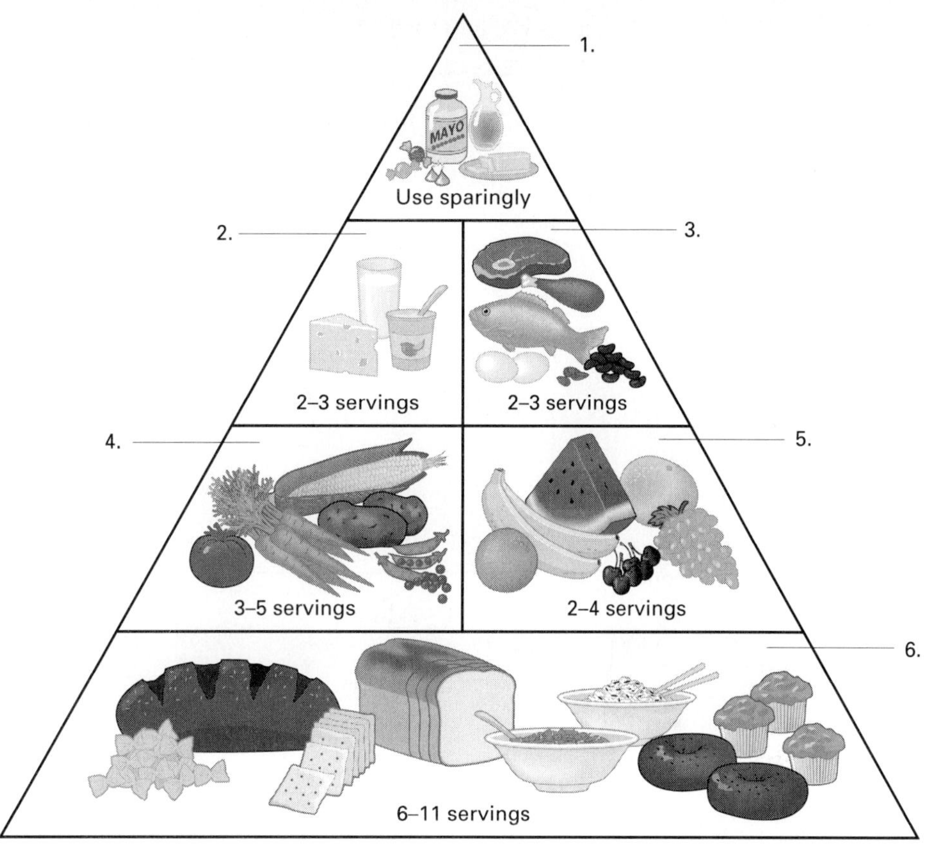

1. _______________________   4. _______________________

2. _______________________   5. _______________________

3. _______________________   6. _______________________

Vocabulary Activity

The following crossword puzzle contains terms that are found in this chapter. Use the clues below to complete the puzzle.

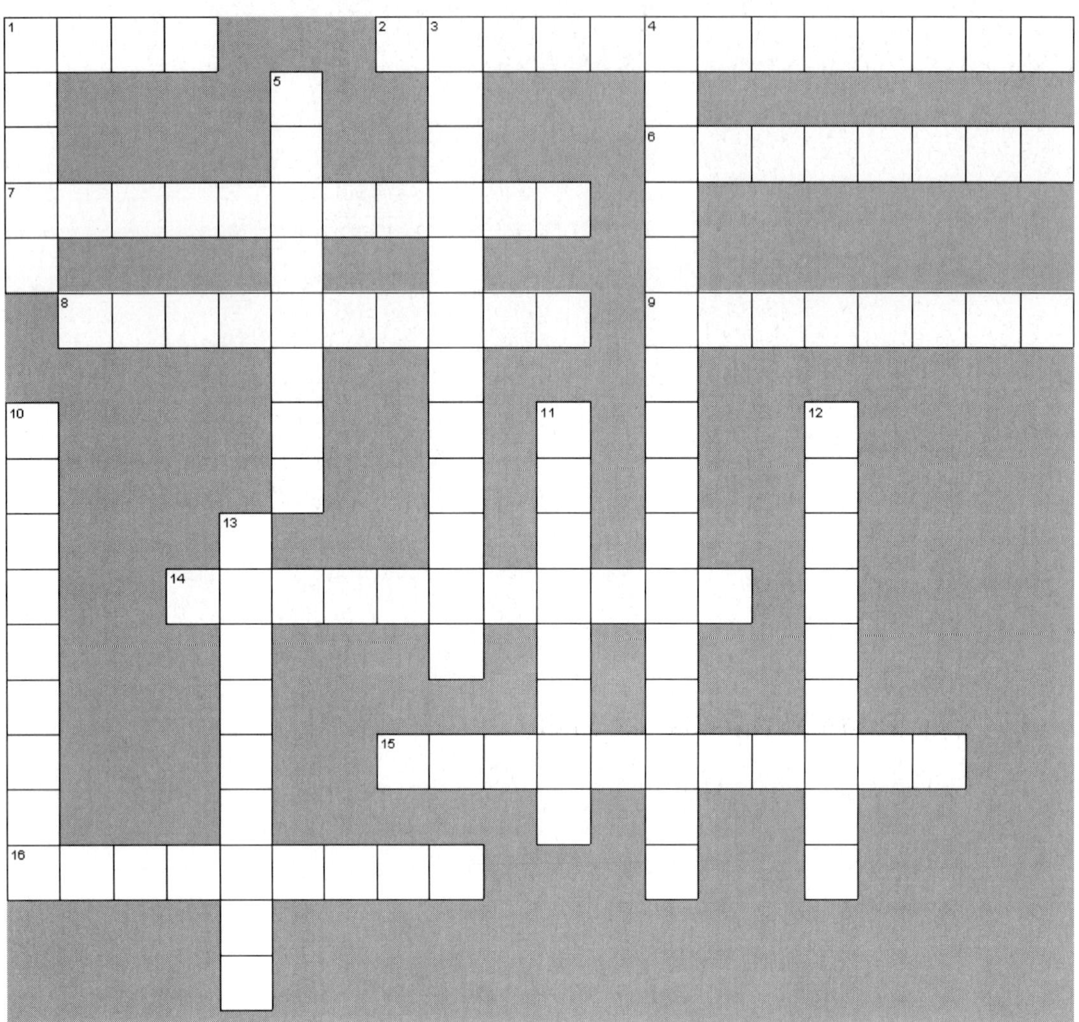

ACROSS

1. one of the major food categories that is a concentrated form of energy
2. one of the three major food categories, including simple sugars, pasta, rice, and other starches
6. one of the three major food categories necessary for rebuild and repair
7. excretion of wastes from the body
8. the process by which broken-down nutrients pass into the bloodstream to be utilized
9. organic compounds that assist in the regulation of certain body processes including the building of tissue
14. profuse sweating
15. fatlike substance that circulates through the body as a lipoprotein
16. substances in food sources that are of value to body functions

DOWN

1. the indigestible carbohydrate component of food
3. the sum of physical and chemical changes, and food transformations that take place in the body
4. the toxic state reached when fat-soluble vitamins are taken in very large quantities
5. the onset of menstruation
10. a collective process of taking in food and using it for proper body functions
11. inorganic elements that regulate fluid and assist in various body functions
12. a thin, yellowy breast liquid that provides an immense amount of immune protection
13. the breakdown of food achieved both mechanically and chemically

Developing Vocabulary

Writing Practice

Beside each word below, write a complete sentence using the word. For each sentence, check for accuracy of content, spelling, and punctuation.

1. carbohydrates _______________________________

____

____

2. digestion _______________________________

____

____

3. assimilation _______________________________

____

____

4. absorption _______________________________

____

____

5. hypervitaminosis _______________________________

____

____

6. proteins_______________________________

____

____

7. vitamins _______________________________

____

____

8. minerals _______________________________

____

____

True or False

If the definition on the right corresponds to the word on the left, then check True, if the word and definition do not correspond, check False.

TRUE   FALSE   WORD

____   ____   1. **Fiber:** the indigestible carbohydrate component of food

____   ____   2. **Digestion:** the breakdown of food achieved both mechanically and chemically

____   ____   3. **Carbohydrates:** one of the three major food categories, including simple sugars, pasta, rice, and other starches

____   ____   4. **Assimilation:** inorganic elements that regulate fluid and assist in various body functions

____   ____   5. **Nutrition:** a collective process of taking in food and using it for proper body functions

Spell Correctly

In each of the sets of words below, one word is spelled correctly. Circle the correctly spelled word.

1.   a. menrache   c. mearcae
      b. menarche   d. manarche

2.   a. colostmum   c. colostrum
      b. colastrum   d. colustrum

3.   a. diaphoresis   c. diaphoresos
      b. daiphoresis   d. diapheresis

4.   a. cholesterol   c. chlesteorl
      b. cholasterol   d. cholhsterol

5.   a. nutriints   c. nutrieets
      b. nutreints   d. nutrients

Practice Scenario(s)

After reading this chapter in the text, read the following scenario(s) and answer the questions following each of them.

Situation 1

Nancy Gallagher is a 23-year-old who has come to the ER for possible fecal impaction. She has not had a bowel movement in 10 days. Nancy states that prior to the constipation, she had diarrhea with ribbon-like stools for three weeks. She says that this has been her bowel habit for the past two years. She is complaining of nausea and belching. Bowel sounds are present in all four quadrants, but her abdomen is distended. The physician orders an enema, which provides relief, and diagnoses her with irritable bowel syndrome.

1. What is your understanding of irritable bowel syndrome?

____

____

____

2. What diet will probably be ordered for Ms. Gallagher?

____

____

____

3. What foods are included in a high fiber diet?

____

____

____

4. What is refined sugar?

____

____

____

Situation 2

Mr. Kilgallan is suffering from malnutrition secondary to metastatic CA. Mr. Kilgallan is edentulous and has difficulty with solid food.

1. What kind of diet will probably be prescribed for Mr. Kilgallan?

____

____

____

2. How might Mr. Kilgallan's diet be modified?

____

____

____

Situation 3

Mrs. Smith has been diagnosed with severe hypertension and athero-sclerosis. Her cholesterol level is 400.

1. What dietary modifications might the physician prescribe?

____

____

____

2. What foods should Mrs. Smith avoid?

____

____

____

Situation 4

Mrs. Fischer is a 47-year-old mother of three who has decided it is time to lose weight. She is being followed by home care after a right total knee replacement. She is 5 foot, 4 inches, and 260 pounds. The doctor wants her to lose 100 pounds.

1. How many pounds are safe to lose per week?

____

____

____

2. How many calories must she cut out each week in order to lose two pounds?

____

____

____

3. How many calories should her daily intake be?

____

____

____

Chapter 19

Care Delivery
for the Whole Person

Chapter Review

Multiple Choice

1. The physical changes of the human body are referred to as
   a. development.
   b. growth.
   c. biology.
   d. physiology.

2. Safety and security needs are satisfied by
   a. shelter and clothing.
   b. oxygen and food.
   c. love and respect.
   d. praise and regard.

3. Which theorist developed a stage theory of human growth and development?
   a. Maslow
   b. Shelly
   c. Erikson
   d. Mitchinson

4. Learning to walk, talk, and perform tasks independently helps the toddler to gain a sense of
   a. autonomy.
   b. trust.
   c. initiative.
   d. industry.

5. Erikson describes adolescence as the stage of
   a. industry vs. inferiority.
   b. intimacy vs. isolation.
   c. initiative vs. guilt.
   d. identity vs. role confusion.

6. Masters and Johnson described the human sexual response in phases which include all except
   a. excitement.
   b. plateau.
   c. recovery.
   d. guilt.

7. Which theorist believed that sexuality is rooted in the unconscious mind?
   a. Masters
   b. Johnson
   c. Erikson
   d. Freud

8. As a CCA, you responsibilities regarding a patient's sexuality involve
   a. responding to sexual expression with judgement.
   b. encouraging concerns to be directed to the nurse.
   c. avoiding questions about sexual problems.
   d. discouraging discussion of sexual issues.

9. What helps an infant to gain a sense of trust?
   a. negative feedback
   b. consistent nurturing
   c. intermittent reinforcement
   d. sexual stimulation

10. Which of the following statements is not true regarding the spirituality of your clients?
    a. Religious disclosure is optional.
    b. Practices should be discouraged.
    c. Clergymen must be available.
    d. Beliefs can be supported.

11. What factor does NOT affect one's traditions and beliefs?
    a. ethnicity
    b. culture
    c. religion
    d. generativity

12. When care for a toddler, the CCA should do all of the following except
    a. offer praise for accomplishments.
    b. encourage parents to sleep over.
    c. permit child to explore equipment.
    d. choose age-specific toys.

13. Which of the following would not demonstrate regard for the age-specific needs of the adolescent patient?
    a. include teen in decisions
    b. encourage socialization with peers
    c. provide privacy during procedures
    d. inform parents of all conversations

Identification Exercise

Label the figure below:

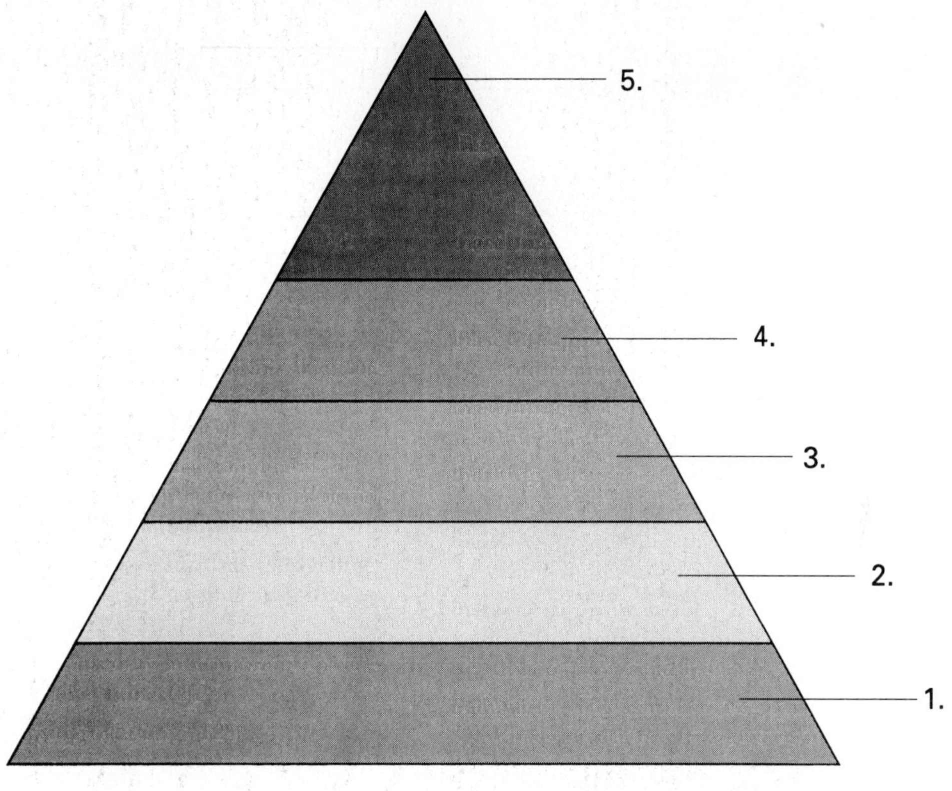

1.________________________

2.________________________

3.________________________

4.________________________

5.________________________

Vocabulary Activity

The following crossword puzzle contains terms that are found in this chapter. Use the clues below to complete the puzzle.

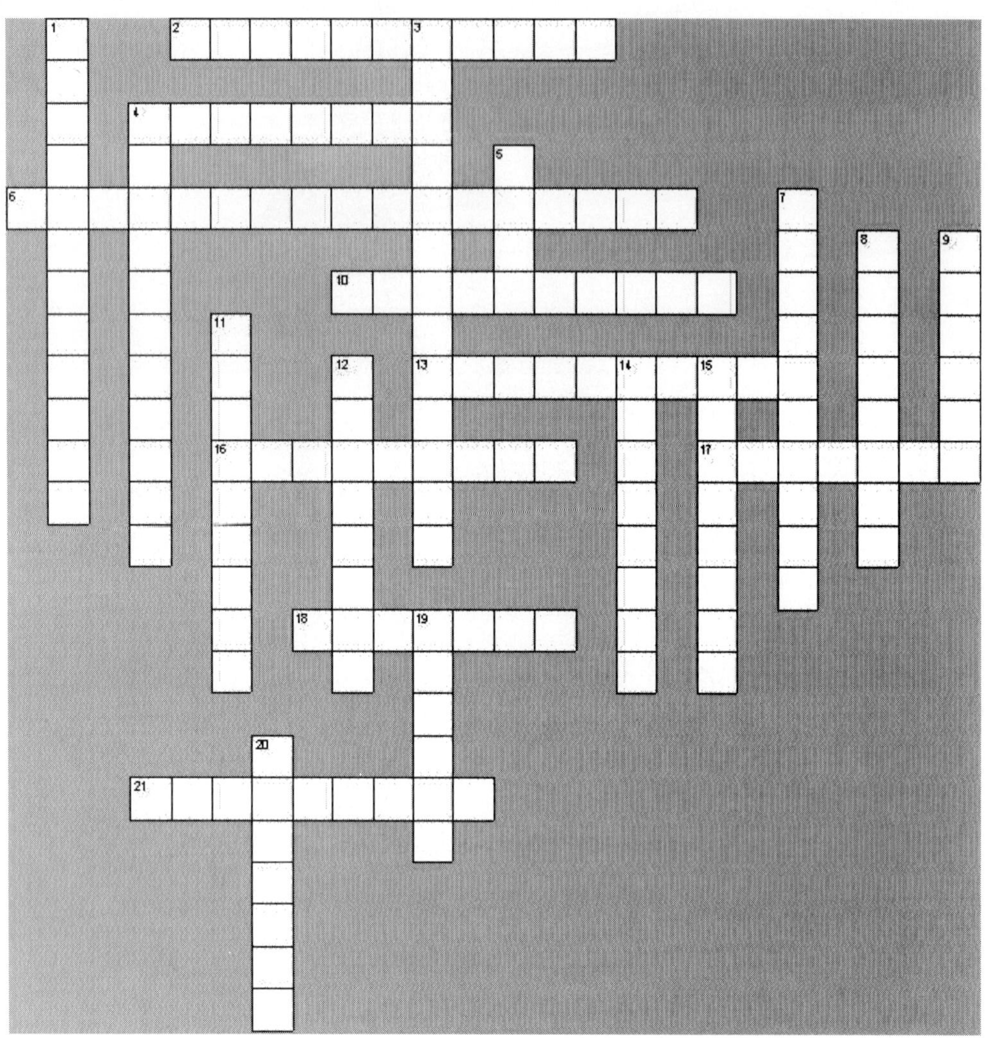

ACROSS

2. growth to full size or maturity
4. distinguishing character or personality of an individual
6. quest to find one's identity, the purpose of life and one's existence
10. internal value and worth recognized by oneself
13. having the power of originating or producing; not self-focused
16. groups of people within a cultural system who are given special status based on religion, language, etc.
17. to lose all hope of confidence
18. marked aversion aroused by something highly distasteful
21. collective characterics that mark the differences between male and female

DOWN

1. accomplishments and learning of a life stage
3. basic needs that include water, food, and oxygen
4. of lower or lower degree of rank
5. sexual intercourse without consent chiefly by force or deception
7. returning behaviorally to an earlier stage of development
8. to start certain activities
9. sex of an individual
11. quality of state of being complete or undivided
12. one who holds the view that any ultimate reality is unknown
14. self-directed and able to do for oneself
15. state of working to achieve a goal
19. physical changes of the human body throughout the life span
20. mores of a people that separates them from others

Developing Vocabulary

Writing Practice

Beside each word below, write a complete sentence using the word. For each sentence, check for accuracy of content, spelling, and punctuation.

1. gender ____

____

____

2. rape ____

____

____

3. self-actualization _____________________________________

____

____

4. competencies ____

____

____

5. inferiority ____

____

____

6. agnostic____

____

____

7. generative____

____

____

8. self-esteem ____

____

____

True or False

If the definition on the right corresponds to the word on the left, then check True, if the word and definition do not correspond, check False.

TRUE   FALSE   WORD

____   ____   1. **Self-actualization:** internal value and worth recognized by oneself

____   ____   2. **Industry:** the state of working to achieve a goal

____   ____   3. **Development:** to start certain activities

____   ____   4. **Disgust:** the collective characteristics that mark the differences between male and female

____   ____   5. **Regression:** the accomplishments and learning of a life stage

Spell Correctly

In each of the sets of words below, one word is spelled correctly. Circle the correctly spelled word.

1. a. despiar   c. dispair
    b. despoir   d. despair

2. a. competencees   c. competenceis
    b. competencies   d. competincies

3. a. physiologicol c. physoilogical
    b. physiological d. physyological

4. a. igtegrity   c. integrity
    b. intugrity   d. inetgrity

5. a. ethnicety   c. ethnicaty
    b. ethnacity   d. ethnicity

Practice Scenario(s)

After reading this chapter in the text, read the following scenario(s) and answer the questions following each of them.

Situation 1

Mrs. Jones is a 40-year-old woman who had a total hysterectomy due to ovarian cancer. She is married and has three children. Two days post-op she tells you that she is "no longer a woman." What will you say?

____

____

____

____

Situation 2

Tim Morgan is a 17 year old who is a resident in a rehabilitation center. He was admitted for injuries resulting from an automobile accident. He has paraplegia as a result of the accident. He is visited often by friends. One night you find him and a girlfriend in bed together. You do not know what they have been doing, but you are upset by this, and you tell her to leave immediately and that you are going to tell his mother what you saw. If you could replay this scenario, how would you replay it, and why?

____

____

____

____

Situation 3

Mr. and Mrs. Snow are residents in the LTC where you work. They share a private room, are happy, and enjoy time alone together. One night, you forget to knock on the door before you enter, and you see them naked in bed together. What should you do?

____

____

____

____

Situation 4

Jane Ruccocas is a three-year-old patient in the pediatric unit. She is playing with a doll and talking to the doll about touching her "privates." She starts to get angry with the doll and throws it on the floor saying, "Jane's a bad girl and needs to be punished." What do you do?

Situation 5

Harvey Sherr is a 56-year-old patient who is being discharged from the inpatient psychiatric unit. He has been treated for depression and seems ready for discharge. While you are helping him pack his bags, he says, "You are such a kind person, and you helped me so much." He tells you he finds you attractive and that he would like to see you after he has returned home. What will you say?

Situation 6

A physician asks you to assist with a therapeutic abortion, but you are opposed because of religious convictions. What would you do?

Situation 7

Mrs. Wisneski lives in a rundown row house in a changing neighborhood. At 79 years old, she is afraid to walk to the corner store to pick up groceries. Many times, she goes without necessary food because of this fear. In addition, Mrs. Wisneski's plumbing requires major repair, but she doesn't have the finances to fix it.

1. At what level is Mrs. Wisneski in Maslow's Hierarchy?

____

____

____

2. Why is this important?

____

____

____

Situation 8

Consider Mr. Thomas, a 38-year-old married man with two children. He is admitted to the hospital with the diagnosis of ulcerative colitis. He is afraid to eat because each time he does he has episodes of diarrhea, which are painful and disruptive to his work routine. (He is an electrician and works at your hospital.) Mr. Thomas is put on a low-residue diet and medications to help him control his diarrhea and meet his nutritional needs. He is then discharged from the hospital. When he returns to work, he is told that his job will be phased out within the month. He needs to find a new job to support his family. He tries to save money by not purchasing his costly prescriptions. He finds a new job in six weeks and is able to purchase his prescriptions again. His wife has also found employment, as a secretary to the district attorney of the county. She is working long hours with her boss and is often busy. She seems to be more interested in her job than in her husband and two children. Mr. Thomas becomes depressed because of this, and he stops caring for his ulcerative colitis. He goes to visit the doctor because he has blood in his stool. When the doctor asks him what is happening in his life, he says, "Why bother caring for myself; my wife doesn't love me any more."

1. When he is not eating properly because of the painful episodes of diarrhea, at what level of need (according to Maslow's pyramid) is Mr. Thomas' focus?

____

____

____

2. When Mr. Thomas learns that he needs to find a new job, what concern will Mr. Thomas now confront on this pyramid of needs?

____

____

____

3. When Mr. Thomas says that his wife doesn't love him anymore, what level of need is unfulfilled for Mr. Thomas?

____

____

____

Care Delivery for the Dying Patient

Chapter Review

Multiple Choice

1. Who is credited with describing the stages of death and dying?
   a. Ross
   b. Freud
   c. Maslow
   d. Erikson

2. The stages of death and dying include all but
   a. denial.
   b. bargaining.
   c. regression.
   d. depression.

3. What legal document ensures that advanced directives will be discussed with patients?
   a. Omnibus Budget Reconciliation Act
   b. Mental Health Law of 1979
   c. Patient Self Determination Act
   d. Advanced Directive Law

4. A surrogate decision maker's role begins when the individual who designated this decision maker becomes
   a. terminal.
   b. bankrupt.
   c. aphasic.
   d. unconscious.

5. Which stage of death and dying depicts the client as refusing to accept the diagnosis?
   a. bargaining
   b. depression
   c. regression
   d. denial

6. Which of the following is a type of advanced directive?
   a. living will
   b. attorney in fact
   c. surrogate document
   d. durable attorney

7. Which of the following is NOT true regarding hospice?
   a. begins with hospital discharge
   b. offers support to families
   c. employs respite volunteers
   d. provides holistic care

8. Who determines that an individual is incapacitated?
   a. attorney in fact
   b. physician
   c. judge
   d. surrogate decision maker

9. Which type of advanced directive does NOT require designating a surrogate decision maker?
   a. attorney in fact
   b. living will
   c. self determination
   d. durable power of attorney

10. The inability to recognize, comprehend, and weigh the risks of alternative treatment options defines
    a. competent.
    b. incapacitated.
    c. incarcerated.
    d. committed.

11. Death with dignity encourages all BUT
    a. pain management.   c. holistic treatment.
    b. hospice care.   d. natural death.

12. The decision NOT to honor an advanced directive requires the assistance of the
    a. ethics committee.   c. medical review board.
    b. primary physician.   d. QA task force.

13. The decision to divide $5,000,000 equally among four family members to pay for health care costs illustrates
    a. autonomy.   c. beneficence.
    b. distribution.   d. non-maleficence.

14. Which of the following is NOT true regarding ethical dilemmas?
    a. choices aren't absolute
    b. decisions are multilevel
    c. risks are weighed
    d. benefits aren't factored

Vocabulary Activity

The following word search puzzle contains terms that are found in this chapter. Use the word list below to locate the hidden words in the grid.

```
S X N U F R Z Z L N N S T S L S C U D J M Z H Z I
Y U I L I V I N G W I L L G I Z D S R W I G O I K
Y X R N N K U W A M V O Q E R U G A G Z N D S J J
A K W R C Y S B D Q H O E K N D S O Q Z S E P O W
O C M X O A F O V X D K N O D W Z O Y C D Q I H A
E V O D M G P N A T T O R N E Y - I N - F A C T R
I H G V P V A A N G E R W H A M L V U Y O W E B J
C C P C E V K T C O G G U S T G L P N O G W N A V
F W N R T R E H E I W V O D H Z E J O T D B I N L
G E O V E R T Q D D T I Q E W U S X F I F D A O L
G C G G N Y O H D K E A Z P I V O J Q P C P K O U
J X C X T E M R I T K C T R T Q I W H L V M X N P
J V M F T T N Y R C A G I E H K C W Y X S E L T A
V S C F K H M G E S Y J S S D M V Z R D F R E Q I
T N C C I I V V C E B B A S I D Q B A E Q A Y U G
A M M A C C E P T A N C E I G O Q V B A D V B C H
I B A R G A I N I N G J M O N W N M I M K F Q E M
E P G Y Y L Z Q V L G D E N I A L M O B U G H V U
S E L F - D E T E R M I N A T I O N A C T V X K Y
D H N W S I S L H J X E H D Y S E D Z K S I D X B
D U R A B L E P O W E R O F A T T O R N E Y C M Q
Y A J G L E T P D U Z A C O N N F R C Z W R P A L
A M B W B M J I W Z G S M I P I M L E V F U R C B
T X T H J M I L V W B E O N E J E U H U N K A Q P
A F K V Q A B O W H K S T W R N S F U I J R I X R
```

1. acceptance
2. advance directive
3. anger
4. attorney in fact
5. bargaining
6. competent
7. covert
8. death with dignity
9. denial
10. depression

11. durable power of attorney
12. ethical dilemma
13. hospice
14. incapacitated
15. incompetent
16. living will
17. overt
18. self-determination act
19. surrogate decision maker

Developing Vocabulary

Writing Practice

Beside each word below, write a complete sentence using the word. For each sentence, check for accuracy of content, spelling, and punctuation.

1. surrogate __________________________________

____

____

2. bargaining ________________________________

____

____

3. incapacitated ______________________________

____

____

4. covert ____________________________________

____

____

5. incompetent________________________________

____

____

6. dilemma __________________________________

____

____

7. acceptance ________________________________

____

____

8. ethical ____________________________________

____

____

True or False

If the definition on the right corresponds to the word on the left, then check True, if the word and definition do not correspond, check False.

TRUE   FALSE   WORD

_____   _____   1. **Durable power of attorney:** a document appointing a specific person as the surrogate decision maker

_____   _____   2. **Covert:** conflict and debate about the welfare of patients

_____   _____   3. **Self-determination Act:** law sanctioning advance directives, durable powers of attorney, and living wills

_____   _____   4. **Advance directive:** a legal document stating an individual's treatment decisions and designating a surrogate decision maker

_____   _____   5. **Bargaining:** responding to death by making promises or deals with Gods

Spell Correctly

In each of the sets of words below, one word is spelled correctly. Circle the correctly spelled word.

1.   a. incampetent   c. incempetent
      b. incompitent   d. incompetent

2.   a. surrogute   c. surrogote
      b. surrogate   d. surregate

3.   a. dilimma   c. dilemma
      b. dalemma   d. dileema

4.   a. ovirt   c. ovvrt
      b. overt   d. ovret

5.   a. incapacetated   c. incapacitated
      b. incapacutated   d. incapacatated

Practice Scenario(s)

After reading this chapter in the text, read the following scenario(s) and answer the questions following each of them.

Situation 1

Mr. Fiore was just diagnosed with cancer of the pancreas. He feels fine and does not believe the physician who says he has less than six weeks to live. He refuses home care. Mr. Fiore's skin and sclera turn yellow two weeks after his diagnosis. He tells his wife that the doctor poisoned him with that biopsy test he was given.

Mrs. Fiore calls your home care agency and asks for activation. She is frightened by her husband's change of status. She says she has not slept since the diagnosis was pronounced, and she has done nothing but cry. She begs for help. Mr. Fiore has a home evaluation, and, as a result, home care is activated.

When you arrive for personal care assistance, Mr. Fiore asks, "What is cancer of the pancreas?" You assist Mr. Fiore into the shower and tell him you will be right outside the door, changing his bed linens. You overhear Mr. Fiore crying and saying, "Please God, I promise to be a better husband to Mary if you just let me live." When Mr. Fiore gets out of the shower, he is crying and asks you to pray for him. He tells you that he is too young to die.

You have finished with Mr. Fiore's personal care. As you are leaving, Mrs. Fiore corners you at the door. She grabs your arm and begs you not to leave. She is holding you very tightly, and tears are in her eyes. You finally leave the Fiore home. You have spent two hours there, but it felt like two days. You have three more clients to visit today.

1. When Mr. Fiore does not believe the physician and refuses home care, what stage of death and dying is he exhibiting?

   ____

   ____

   ____

2. When Mr. Fiore believes that the doctor poisoned him with the biopsy test, what stage of death and dying is Mr. Fiore exhibiting?

   ____

   ____

   ____

3. What do you say when Mr. Fiore asks you "What is cancer of the pancreas?"

   ____

   ____

   ____

4. What stage of death and dying is Mr. Fiore exhibiting when he is crying and pleading to God to let him live and promising to be a better husband?

   ____

   ____

   ____

5. How will you respond when Mr. Fiore cries and asks you to pray for him and says that he is too young to die?

   ____

   ____

   ____

   ____

6. What will you do when Mrs. Fiore grabs your arm and begs you not to leave?

   ____

   ____

   ____

7. Since you feel drained of your energy when you leave the Fiore home, what can you do to replenish your drained energy?

   ____

   ____

   ____

Understanding Mental Illness

Chapter Review

Multiple Choice

1. What is NOT true about a psychotic patient?
   a. hears imaginary voices
   b. lives in distorted thinking.
   c. displays peculiar emotions.
   d. questions inappropriate perceptions.

2. The term that literally means "split mind" is
   a. megalomania.
   b. schizophrenia.
   c. dysthymia.
   d. nihilism.

3. The delusion in which a person holds to a false belief of exaggerated power, status, or beauty is
   a. tactile.
   b. persecutory.
   c. grandeur.
   d. nihilistic.

4. Which of the following is NOT a symptom of schizophrenia?
   a. visual hallucination
   b. delusion of grandeur
   c. flat affect
   d. pressured speech

5. The personality disorder characterized by unstable moods, intense and unstable relationships, and "splitting" is
   a. antisocial.
   b. avoidant.
   c. histrionic.
   d. borderline.

6. The mood disorder whose symptoms include severe episodes of mania and depression is
   a. bipolar.
   b. delusional.
   c. dysthymic.
   d. cyclothymic.

7. The defense mechanism defined as making up for a weakness in on aspect of life by excelling at another is
   a. suppression.
   b. compensation.
   c. displacement.
   d. projection.

8. Refusing to own something you did emotionally and blaming another for it is called
   a. displacement.
   b. projection.
   c. compensation.
   d. regression.

9. The anxiety disorder characterized by an intense and irrational fear is termed __________ disorder.
   a. dissociative
   b. anxiety
   c. phobic
   d. panic

10. Alzheimer's disease is a form of
    a. delirium.
    b. dementia.
    c. psychosis.
    d. neurosis.

11. Criteria for a mental retardation diagnosis includes all BUT
    a. IQ is less than 80.
    b. adaptation to environment is difficult.
    c. delirium and dementia coexist.
    d. symptoms are present before 18 years of age.

12. All of the following symptoms must be exhibited for a diagnosis of clinical depression except
    a. chronic insomnia.
    b. weight fluctuation.
    c. daily sadness.
    d. irrational fear.

13. Which is NOT true about delirium?
    a. causes confusion.
    b. appears suddenly.
    c. produces disorientation.
    d. progresses slowly.

14. Neuroses cause all the symptoms below except
    a. persistent fear.
    b. irrational belief.
    c. marked anxiety.
    d. compulsive acts.

Vocabulary Activity

The following word search puzzle contains terms that are found in this chapter. Use the word list below to locate the hidden words in the grid.

```
I M O L T S J J J A H C W K D U H K Y U
V T W D I S S O C I A T I V E A D O T E
S A N T I S O C I A L I T D P S T I D E
S C H I Z O I D G H L R H B E F O H Y I
O P H O D E L I R I U M D R N Y V O C E
S A D I S T I C J D C P R N D S B O Y H
M T B H Z O M U O Z I S A W E N A V O O
P S Y C H O S I S E N Q W L N B F D I L
W M R S D K P L D T A K A N C K O X V K
S N F E I C J H R J T Y L J E U P B T C
Q Q G B O R D E R L I N E Y L R A O I V
O C O G N I T I V E O L C U A S R U N B
Y P H Y P E R S O M N I A U P I A C S H
J W G N E U R O S I S I T C N H N I O N
T L F H F L A T O L E R A N C E O M M W
P R U V Q X X A N X I E T Y I O I R N R
G H W J L P D E L U S I O N Q M A N I A
B U I C L R N L D E M E N T I A B H A A
X Q O T L P U P P H O B I A V K I F A H
B H L R K B A A H I I W A S U W D W A Q
```

1. antisocial	14. hypersomnia
2. anxiety	15. insomnia
3. borderline	16. mania
4. catatonia	17. neurosis
5. cognitive	18. paranoia
6. delirium	19. phobia
7. delusion	20. psychosis
8. dementia	21. sadistic
9. dependence	22. schizoid
10. dissociative	23. schizophrenia
11. euphoria	24. tolerance
12. flat	25. withdrawal
13. hallucinations	

Developing Vocabulary

Writing Practice

Beside each word below, write a complete sentence using the word. For each sentence, check for accuracy of content, spelling, and punctuation.

1. withdrawal ________________________________

   ____

   ____

2. insomnia ________________________________

   ____

   ____

3. antisocial ________________________________

   ____

   ____

4. tolerance ________________________________

   ____

   ____

5. paranoia ________________________________

   ____

   ____

6. hypersomnia ________________________________

   ____

   ____

7. anxiety ________________________________

   ____

   ____

8. dependence ________________________________

   ____

   ____

True or False

If the definition on the right corresponds to the word on the left, then check True, if the word and definition do not correspond, check False.

TRUE   FALSE   WORD

____   ____   1. **Mania:** an expansive, persistent, elevated or irritable mood that lasts for at least one week

____   ____   2. **Dissociative:** inability to fall or stay asleep

____   ____   3. **Flat:** senility often results from slow, chronic degeneration of brain tissue

____   ____   4. **Cognitive:** pertaining to awareness with reasoning, thinking, and judgment

____   ____   5. **Euphoria:** a sense of well-being often seen in situations of addiction

Spell Correctly

In each of the sets of words below, one word is spelled correctly. Circle the correctly spelled word.

1.   a. delerium   c. dilirium
      b. delirium   d. delireum

2.   a. schizophrenia   c. sphizophrenia
      b. schizophrenua   d. schizophrecia

3.   a. schizoid   c. schizood
      b. schisoid   d. schiziod

4.   a. catatonia   c. catetonia
      b. catattnia   d. catatania

5.   a. hallucinitions   c. hallucinasions
      b. hallucinations   d. hallicinations

Practice Scenario(s)

After reading this chapter in the text, read the following scenario(s) and answer the questions following each of them.

Situation 1

Harry Burns is a 50-year-old who has been admitted to the mental-health inpatient-treatment unit. He is diagnosed with major depression. Mr. Burns is often tearful, awakens early in the morning, eats only a few bites of his meals, moves very slowly, always has a sad affect, and has difficulty falling asleep. He says very little when you talk to him, and he tells you that he is "a sinner and doesn't deserve to live."

One day, you try to start a conversation with Mr. Burns and he says, "I don't have anything interesting to say; just go away." You respond to him in a concerned and caring manner, and he says nothing in response to the few questions that you asked him. You sit with him for 15 minutes, and then you come back again later to see him. This time Mr. Burns is not where you expected to find him. You suspect he is in bed in his room. In a few minutes, Mr. Burns comes to the dinning room where you are waiting. You offer him a seat. He sits down and says, "I'm only here because you want to see me."

The next day Mr. Burns arrives early for your meeting you have scheduled with him. He arrives early for your meeting. He is talkative and tells you that he is feeling "just great." He tells you that you are a wonderful counselor and that he is pleased you expressed an interest in him. He says that he is planning to be discharged as soon as possible and that his employer is awaiting his return to the office. During his conversation, he expresses ideas of interest in investing in the stock market. He also tells you that he was the vice president of an investment firm. He tells you that he is planning a trip to the Bahamas and that he has some women waiting for him on the islands. He has many thoughts that are expressed rapidly and with pressure. His conversation jumps from one topic to the next. In only fifteen minutes of listening to Mr. Burns, you feel exhausted.

Two mornings later, you get a report and find that Mr. Burns' wife visited him and told him that she wants a divorce. You are informed that Mr. Burns does not work for an investment firm and that he is not a vice president. However, his boss did tell him that he could have his job back when he was better. His wife told the nurse that she called two days ago to say that she wanted to visit with him that night. You are told that Mr. Burns is now on a 1:1 observation. You are assigned to do the 1:1. When you relieve the night shift psychiatric technician, he tells you that Mr. Burns did not sleep, that he prayed all-night and cried about his "sins." When you say good morning, Mr. Burns does not respond. When the night shift technician leaves, Mr. Burns says, "I am a worthless loser, and I should be dead."

1. What are the signs and symptoms of major depression?

    ____

    ____

    ____

2. How will you respond when Mr. Burns says: "I don't have anything interesting to say; just go away"?

    ____

    ____

    ____

3. When you suspect that Mr. Burns in bed in his room, what do you do?

    ____

    ____

    ____

4. What do you do with the information Mr. Burns has shared with you about what he has done and what he is going to do?

    ____

    ____

    ____

5. Why would the nurse tell you to do q 15 minute checks and report changes STAT?

    ____

    ____

    ____

6. How do you respond when Mr. Burns says, "I am a worthless loser and I should be dead"?

____

____

____

7. What are the safety precautions of 1:1 observation?

____

____

____

Situation 2

Robert Brady is a 25-year-old male who was admitted four days ago as a resident in the CRR of your Community Mental Health agency. Mr. Brady is helpful to staff and seems healthy and capable. Some of the staff like him, and others think he is untrustworthy. He is a college graduate who recently lost the only job he has held for more than three months. He worked as an accountant for a small firm for 6 months. He was fired from his job when he was accused of sexual harassment and suspected of drug abuse on the job. Mr. Brady refused to submit to a drug test, slapped his supervisor, and ran out of the building. The supervisor pressed charges, and Mr. Brady was ordered by the court to attend mental health outpatient and residential treatment in the community for diagnosis and treatment. His drug screening revealed the presence of cocaine, alcohol, and barbiturates. While visiting, his girlfriend told the staff that he is a liar and he "slaps me around when I won't do what he wants." She also stated that, "He is so persuasive and appealing that I cannot resist him." When she leaves one night, he is sad and says, "I only did drugs when I was depressed. She made me do them."

Mr. Brady does not feel responsible for losing his job or for the problems with his relationship. Mr. Brady is charming with you. He is always telling you how wonderful you are to him. He calls you "the ideal resident counselor." He also tells you how all of the other resident counselors ignore him and that they do not have the same integrity that you have. The psychiatrist who sees Mr. Brady in the outpatient facility diagnoses borderline personality disorder. He grants Mr. Brady an overnight pass.

Mr. Brady goes away for the weekend with his girlfriend. He does not return to the CRR on Sunday night as scheduled. You report this to the oncoming night shift resident counselor. Monday and Tuesday are your scheduled days off. When you return on Wednesday evening, you learn that Mr. Brady returned Monday evening. He spent his unemployment check on the weekend and could not pay his rent. The treatment team is considering discharging him from the CRR if the drug screen results come back positive. Because he was found to be "mentally ill" by the court and ordered to mental health treatment instead of serving jail time for the assault, the team will have to turn his case back to the court. The stipulations of treatment in the CRR were that he remain drug free and abide by all house rules. Before you have time to read the notes in his chart, he approaches you. He is tearful and tells you that he is so happy to see you because "You are the only one who will help me." By the end of your shift, he has convinced you that he should stay in the CRR and that he "made a mistake that won't happen ever again." He expresses thoughts of suicide if he should be "thrown out of the CRR." "I'll kill myself if they want to send me to jail; I need help, not jail." When you tell the other resident counselor on duty about Mr. Brady's thoughts of suicide, he says, "He's faking; he just wants to stay in the community." "Don't take him seriously; he's a typical borderline personality." "He would do something just to scare the staff and to stay out of jail." You are concerned about the real possibility of a suicide attempt even if Mr. Brady wanted just to stay out of jail.

1. Refer to the portion of the scenario where Mr. Brady said, "I only did drugs when I was depressed. She make me do them." What defense mechanism is he using?

2. Mr. Brady does not feel responsible for losing his job or for the problems with his relationship. In what mental health diagnostic category is this a feature?

3. What should you do with all of the information Mr. Brady gives you?

4. Why should you be cautious about your responses and the praise that Mr. Brady gives to you?

____

____

____

5. When Mr. Brady starts talking about killing himself, what behaviors has he used to undermine your therapeutic strategies?

____

____

____

6. What do you do about your concern for this client's safety and the need to respond to such a threat as suicide?

____

____

____

Treating Mental Illness

Chapter Review

Multiple Choice

1. Anxiety can be manifested in all the following ways except
   a. pacing.
   b. worrying.
   c. hallucinating.
   d. chain smoking.

2. The repetition of an act or acts to control anxiety defines
   a. obsession.
   b. depression.
   c. compulsion.
   d. regression.

3. All of the following are management strategies for anxious behavior except
   a. interrupt ritual behaviors.
   b. provide orderly direction.
   c. allow time to respond.
   d. keep client informed.

4. Angry behavior exhibited by a client is all but a
   a. symptom of fear.
   b. sign of frustration.
   c. desire to isolate.
   d. need to control.

5. What tactic should be used to manage hallucinations coupled with hostility?
   a. remove yourself from the area.
   b. let the client act out.
   c. reassure the client he is safe.
   d. demonstrate your fearlessness.

6. An hallucination in which a client tell you she hears God's voice telling her to jump out the window is
   a. tactile.
   b. visual.
   c. auditory.
   d. olfactory.

7. A therapeutic technique for the depressed client might be to
   a. give praise.
   b. avoid silences.
   c. demonstrate sympathy.
   d. question frequently.

8. When a client expresses ideas of suicide, all of the following should be done except
   a. report stat.
   b. question client.
   c. document dialogue.
   d. endorse secrecy.

9. An appropriate intervention for hallucinations is
   a. test the patient's food.
   b. isolate the patient.
   c. sing with the patient.
   d. disagree with the delusion.

10. Which of the following is NOT a type of positive reinforcement?
    a. withhold response.
    b. administer praise.
    c. give attention.
    d. provide food.

11. Reinforcement in which a client is rewarded at the completion of each step is called
    a. intermittent.
    b. negative.
    c. immediate.
    d. end-result.

12. Chaining that teaches a task step by step starting with the first step is termed
    a. end-result.
    b. intermittent.
    c. forward.
    d. negative.

13. A behavior modification technique used to teach social behaviors is
    a. chaining.
    b. shaping.
    c. reinforcement.
    d. baselining.

14. Which statement describes the equation, "Action = benefits obtained risks to be taken?
    a. "Get out of bed to feel better."
    b. "On a scale of 0 to 10, how bad is it?"
    c. "Staying in bed only increases depression."
    d. "If it feels that bad, why get out?"

Vocabulary Activity

The following crossword puzzle contains terms that are found in this chapter. Use the clues below to complete the puzzle.

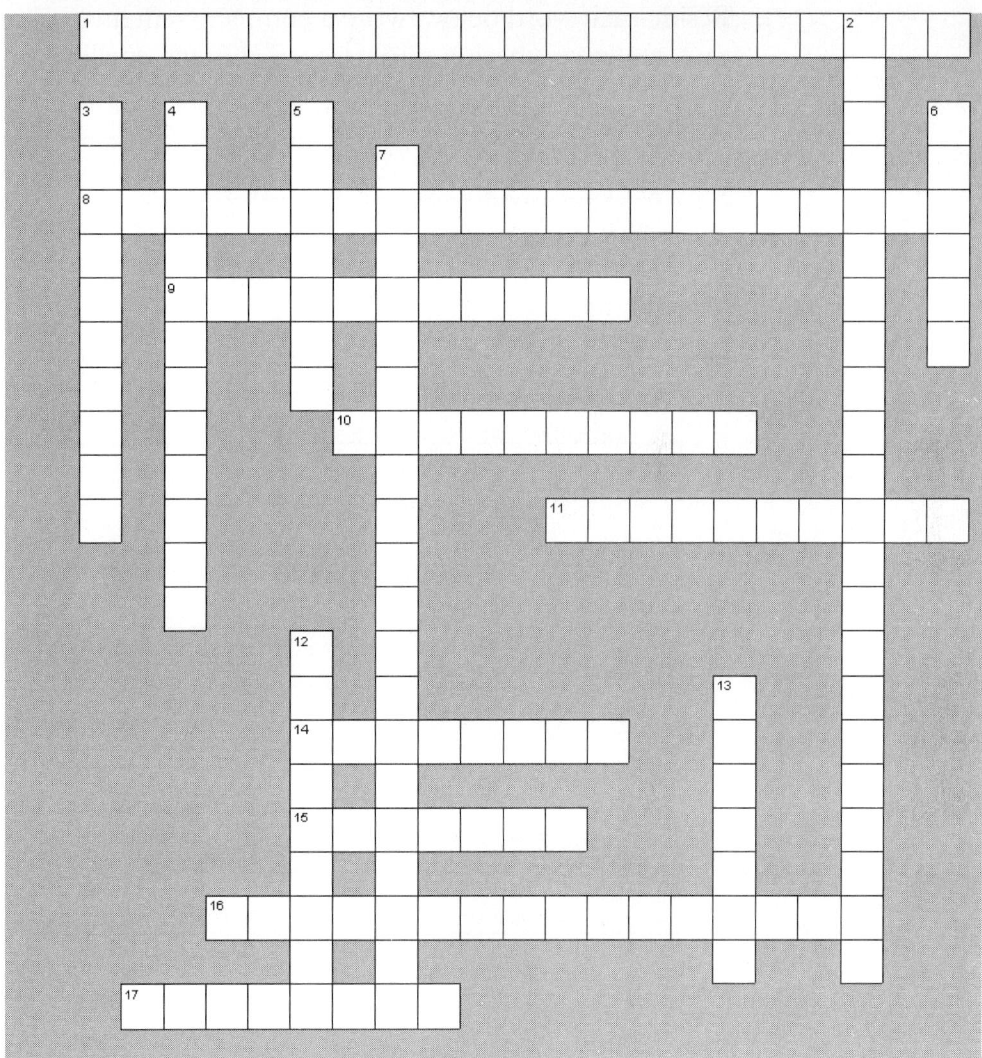

ACROSS

1. strengthening a desired outcome by withholding or punishing when action is not appropriate
8. strengthening of a desired outcome by rewarding the appropriate response
9. inability to make a decision because both sides of the situation seem equal
10. action used to relieve anxiety generated by an obsessive thought
11. analyzing a behavior that requires modification
14. cause of a behavior
15. molding a behavior or teaching the approximate steps of a behavior or task
16. contemplating or entertaining the act of suicide
17. process of teaching a task step-by-step and linking each step together

DOWN

2. reward given at completion of task for strengthening the desired outcome
3. emotional state characterized by extreme sadness, worthlessness, and hopelessness
4. breaking down a procedure into its simplest steps
5. style of passively demanding attention
6. repetition of an act or acts
7. treatment technique that helps reduce undesirable or unwanted behavior
12. persistent and often unreasonable thought that preoccupies one's thought processes
13. generalized feelings of fear and apprehension

Developing Vocabulary

Writing Practice

Beside each word below, write a complete sentence using the word. For
each sentence, check for accuracy of content, spelling, and punctuation.

1. suicidal ideation _______________________________________

____

____

2. whining____

____

____

3. baselining ____

____

____

4. shaping ____

____

____

5. ambivalence ____

____

____

6. chaining ____

____

____

7. end-result reinforcement _____________________________

____

____

8. behavior modification___________________________________

____

____

True or False

If the definition on the right corresponds to the word on the left, then check True, if the word and definition do not correspond, check False.

TRUE   FALSE   WORD

____   ____   1. **Baselining:** strengthening a desired outcome by withholding or punishing when action is not appropriate

____   ____   2. **Behavior modification:** a persistent and often unreasonable thought that preoccupies one's thought processes

____   ____   3. **Stimulus:** the cause of behavior

____   ____   4. **Ritual:** strengthening of a desired outcome by rewarding the appropriate response

____   ____   5. **Task analysis:** breaking down a procedure into its simplest steps

Spell Correctly

In each of the sets of words below, one word is spelled correctly. Circle the correctly spelled word.

1. a. ambivalence   c. ambuvalence
    b. ambivalonce   d. ambivulence

2. a. stimalus   c. stimulus
    b. stemulus   d. stimelus

3. a. compulsion   c. compolsion
    b. compulsian   d. compulsoin

4. a. obsessoin   c. obsession
    b. obsission   d. oisession

5. a. anxaety   c. anxitey
    b. anxiety   d. anxoety

Practice Scenario(s)

After reading this chapter in the text, read the following scenario(s) and answer the questions following each of them.

Situation 1

You are working in a hospital inpatient psychiatric unit. You receive an admission, and the nurse asks you to orient the patient to the unit. As you introduce Mr. Jones to the other patients and show him around, you notice that he mumbles to himself and does not make eye contact with you. He will not allow you to take his blood pressure or height and weight. He says, "Leave me alone, you are not going to touch me, I am the Lord and you want to see me dead." When you say, "Mr Jones, I do not want to see you dead; I want to help you." He responds with, "The voice of the Holy Spirit has told me you want me dead."

Mr. Jones refuses to eat the hospital food because it is poison. It has been two days since admission to the hospital, and he has had only water.

1. When Mr. Jones says to you, "The voice of the Holy Spirit has told me that you want me dead," what distortions of thought and perception is Mr. Jones experiencing?

   ____

   ____

   ____

2. What will you report to the nurse?

   ____

   ____

   ____

3. How would you help to decrease Mr. Jones' suspicions?

   ____

   ____

   ____

4. How might you encourage Mr. Jones to eat?

____

____

____

Situation 2

Martha White is a 24-year-old resident of a community living arrangement. She has been living in this group home for two years. Martha travels every day by public transportation to her vocational workshop. She takes her medication with minimal supervision, and is learning to cook and do laundry.

Her mother visits often and brings her toys, such as dolls. You notice Martha's mother treats Martha as a small child. She talks "baby talk" and does not encourage her daughter to accomplish household chores. She tells you that Martha is just a child and that she will never be able to function as an adult. You know that Martha has mild mental retardation resulting from Down's Syndrome. You are concerned about Martha's treatment plans because each time her mother leaves, it takes a day to get Martha to perform tasks independently again.

The treatment team meets with Martha and her mother to discuss the goals of the rehabilitation plan. Mrs. White tells the team that she is in full agreement and supports the approaches to help Martha become more independent. Nevertheless, the next time Martha's mother visits, she does Martha's laundry and cleans Martha's room for her. Mrs. White says to you, "I know the staff wants her to do these things for herself, but she's my baby." You are assigned to assist Martha in learning to cook scrambled eggs. This is her favorite Sunday breakfast food.

1. When Mrs. White says to you, "I know the staff wants her to do these things for herself, but she's my baby," how will you respond?

____

____

____

2. Regarding your assignment to assist Martha in learning to cook scrambled eggs, what behavior modification teaching method should you use?

____

____

____

C h a p t e r   2 3

Safety and Security Issues in Health Care

Chapter Review

Multiple Choice

1. When a patient acquires an infection during a hospital stay, the infection is referred to as
   a. noncontagious.
   b. airborne.
   c. nosocomial.
   d. droplet.

2. Which principle of body mechanics is violated if a person carries a shoulder bag?
   a. base of support
   b. center of gravity
   c. centrifugal force
   d. force of gravity

3. Which muscles should be used to push, pull or lift heavy objects?
   a. back and gluteals
   b. hamstrings and quadriceps
   c. deltoid and latissimus dorsi
   d. triceps and pectoralis

4. The most important means of preventing the spread of germs is
   a. using a mask.
   b. donning a gown.
   c. washing hands.
   d. wearing gloves.

5. The __________ is the means by which microbes enter the human body.
   a. portal of exit
   b. causative agent
   c. susceptible host
   d. portal of entry

6. The necessary conditions for the growth of every microbe include all but
   a. moisture.
   b. warmth.
   c. darkness.
   d. air.

7. Which of the following procedures requires sterile technique?
   a. bathing a patient.
   b. washing your hands.
   c. catheterizing the bladder.
   d. feeding via gastrostomy.

8. The universal precautions that all health care workers must use to prevent the spread of infection are called __________ precautions.
   a. sterile
   b. standard
   c. contact
   d. aseptic

9. A clinical care associate should wear gloves while
   a. washing hands between patients.
   b. changing a resident's clothing.
   c. changing soiled linens.
   d. serving meal trays.

10. Which isolation precautions require the health care worker to wear an N95 respirator/mask?
    a. droplet
    b. airborne
    c. standard
    d. contact

11. Which isolation precautions are instituted if a patient has MRSA or VRE?
    a. droplet
    b. airborne
    c. contact
    d. enteric

12. When entering the hospital for work, the security officer expects to see the CCA wearing a hospital
    a. lab coat.
    b. uniform.
    c. name tag.
    d. ID badge.

13. What measure must be followed to protect confidentiality of a patient's chart?
    a. Question authorization before releasing chart.
    b. Keep chart in a readily accessible area.
    c. Store chart in patient's room.
    d. Allow chart access to persons in labcoats.

14. With whom should you share your hospital computer password?
    a. coworkers
    b. security
    c. no one
    d. spouse

Vocabulary Activity

The following crossword puzzle contains terms that are found in this chapter. Use the clues below to complete the puzzle.

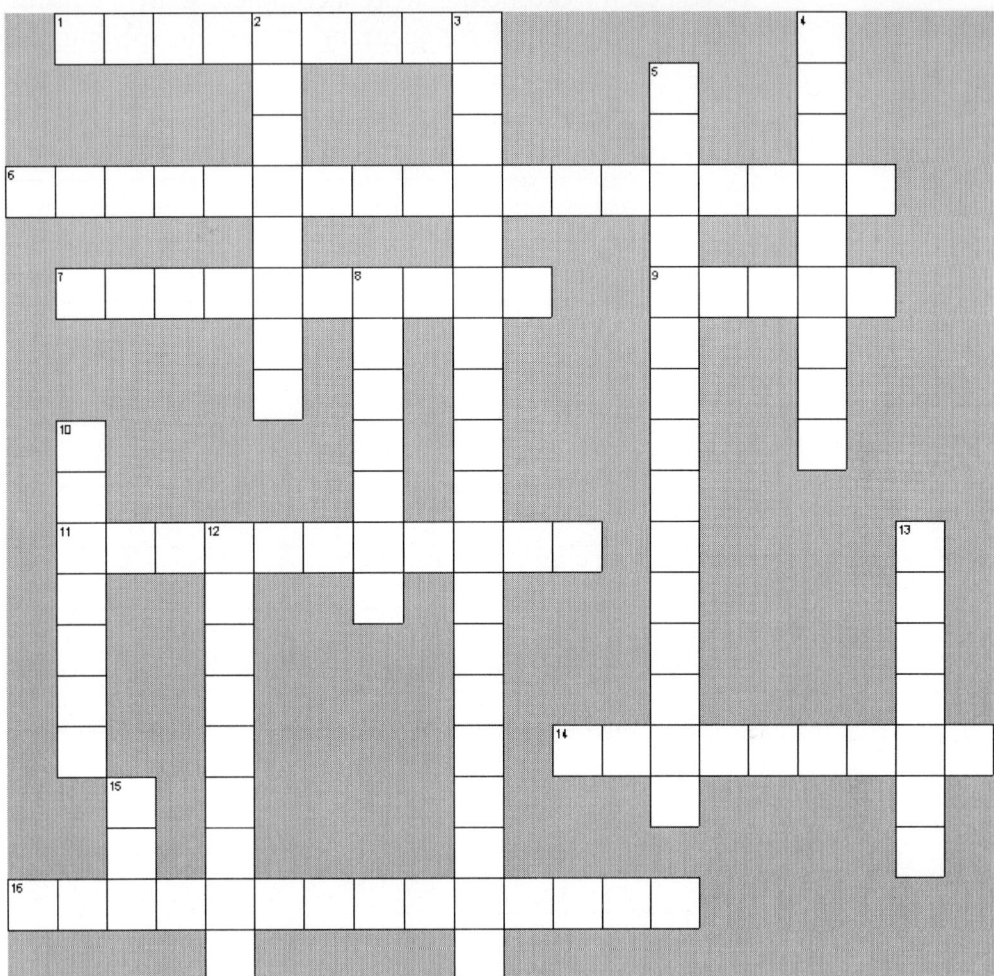

ACROSS

1. disease-producing organisms
6. way microbes are moved or transferred from the reservoir to the susceptible host
7. pertaining to the origin in a health-care facility, such as a hospital-acquired infection
9. bacteria present in the intestines, only harmful when spread to other body orifices
11. immediate daily surroundings of an individual where personal needs are met
14. conditions in which microbes grow
16. small living thing not visible to the naked eye

DOWN

2. openings in the body
3. CDC guidelines that must be followed to prevent the transmission of pathogenic organisms
4. piece of equipment used to sterilize articles using steam under pressure
5. person prime for developing an infectious disease
8. natural center of gravity in the human body
10. free from infection
12. method of caring for persons who have communicable diseases
13. force that creates weight by pulling us down
15. organization who established guidelines for reducing the risk of disease transmission

Developing Vocabulary

Writing Practice

Beside each word below, write a complete sentence using the word. For each sentence, check for accuracy of content, spelling, and punctuation.

1. autoclave ____

____

____

2. isolation ____

____

____

3. asepsis ____

____

____

4. CDC ____

____

____

5. E. coli ____

____

____

6. standard precautions _____________________________________

____

____

7. orifices ____

____

____

8. nosocomial ____

____

____

True or False

If the definition on the right corresponds to the word on the left, then check True, if the word and definition do not correspond, check False.

TRUE	FALSE	WORD
____	____	1. **Autoclave:** openings in the body
____	____	2. **Environment:** the immediate daily surroundings of an individual where personal needs are met
____	____	3. **Midline:** the natural center of gravity in the human body
____	____	4. **Mode of transmission:** conditions in which microbes grow
____	____	5. **Susceptile host:** person prime for developing an infectious disease

Spell Correctly

In each of the sets of words below, one word is spelled correctly. Circle the correctly spelled word.

1. a. reservoir   c. reservior
    b. reservoor   d. reservour

2. a. nosocomial   c. nosocomeal
    b. nosicomial   d. nosocomail

3. a. microorganisms   c. microorgnaisms
    b. mecroorganisms   d. microorgainsms

4. a. aseptis   c. asepsis
    b. asessis   d. aeepsis

5. a. pathogens   c. pathogans
    b. pathogins   d. pathonens

Practice Scenario(s)

After reading this chapter in the text, read the following scenario(s) and answer the questions following each of them.

Situation 1

Imagine yourself riding the bus to work. Notice all the things your hands touch. Think of how many other people have touched those same objects or have sneezed and accidentally sprayed the seat that you sat in. Think about the individuals who coughed into their hands and touched the handle of your office when they stopped in to ask a question. Now, you're ready to eat lunch, a sandwich. You're too rushed and don't wash your hands. Do you know how many germs might enter your mouth? Thank goodness your immune system is strong, and you are healthy. Those microbes, in most cases, will be destroyed. But if you haven't cared for your health, you could become ill. Some microbes will not be destroyed in spite of your healthy state. Hepatitis A virus is highly infectious, and food handlers who do not wash their hands after using the bathroom can spread this virus to healthy individuals. Identify each link in the chain of infection in this scenario.

____

____

____

____

Situation 2

A hamburger is undercooked. You eat it and develop the infection salmonella, a type of food poisoning. Identify each link in the chain of infection.

____

____

____

____

Situation 3

Chicken pox is a disease caused by the herpes virus varicella, an airborne virus. You've never had the disease, but then your son develops chicken pox, and so do you. Why did this occur?

____

____

____

____

Situation 4

You are assigned to help Mr. Jamal transfer from his bed to a chair. Mr. Jamal is paraplegic and weighs 210 lbs. What principles of body mechanics must you employ to ensure your safety and Mr. Jamal's safety?

____

____

____

____

The Client's Care Environment

Chapter Review

Multiple Choice

1. Some reasons for Medicare nursing home admission include all except
   a. need for rehabilitation.
   b. desire for safety.
   c. lack of caregivers.
   d. necessity for skilled care.

2. What law ensures individualized care and resident rights for persons who live in a nursing home?
   a. Patient Self Determination Act
   b. Omnibus Budget Reconciliation Act
   c. Quality of Life Act
   d. Patient Bill of Rights Act

3. What title is used to refer to individuals who live in a long-term care facility?
   a. patient
   b. client
   c. customer
   d. resident

4. During daytime hours and for social activities and meals, individuals who live in a nursing home usually wear
   a. hospital gowns.
   b. night gowns.
   c. personal clothes.
   d. incontinence briefs.

5. What resident information is not necessary to provide individualized care?
   a. former lifestyle
   b. family dynamics
   c. personal dislikes
   d. political affiliation

6. Risk factors for falls include all except
    a. unstable gait.
    b. visual impairment.
    c. unfamiliar environment.
    d. loss of self esteem.

7. Which of the following is not a true statement about restraints?
    a. Side rails are considered restraints.
    b. Restraints prevent falls and injury.
    c. Residents have the right to be restraint free.
    d. Complications of restraints are lethal.

8. What measure must be followed if a patient is placed in any type of restraint?
    a. A doctor's order must be written.
    b. Staff members must check every two hours.
    c. Restraints must be released every 15 minutes.
    d. A nurse must assess the resident daily.

9. Which of the following is a possible cause of goal-directed wandering among residents?
    a. recent confusion
    b. searching for someone
    c. need to remain busy
    d. former lifestyle

10. Staff should intervene with a resident's wandering behavior when it
    a. annoys staff.   c. encourages mobility.
    b. interferes with safety.   d. promotes contentment.

11. If you find unsafe living conditions while working as a home health aide, you should
    a. repair the problem.
    b. call a repair service.
    c. report to your supervisor.
    d. suggest low-cost contacts.

12. Alternatives to restraints include all of the following except
    a. close supervision.
    b. wander alarms.
    c. locked tray chairs.
    d. verbal distraction.

13. Which measure reduces a patient's risk of falling?
    a. elevated siderails.   c. adequate lighting.
    b. locked Geri chairs.   d. safety belts.

14. Which of the following is not a possible complication of restraints?
    a. incontinence   c. hepatitis
    b. death   d. fractures

Identification Exercise

Label the figure below:

Typical Patient Unit

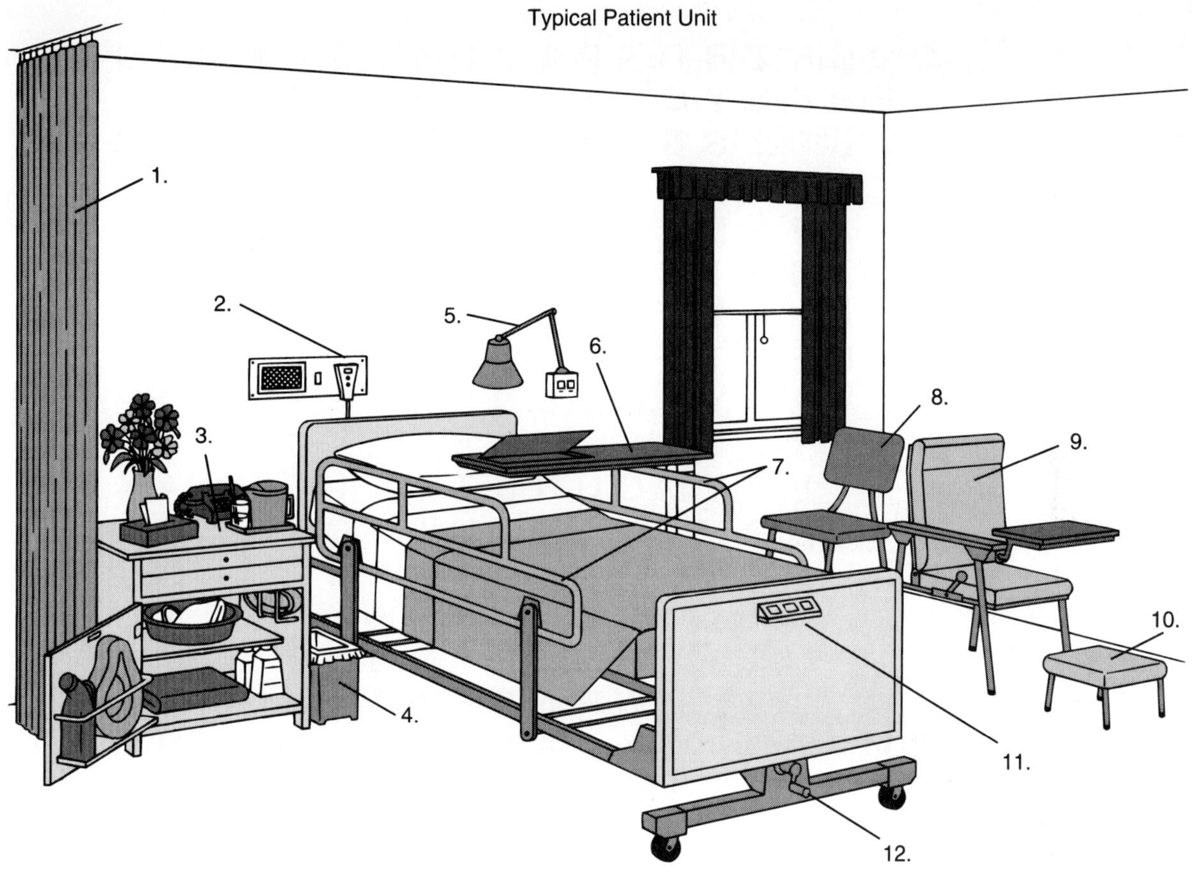

1. _________________	7. _________________
2. _________________	8. _________________
3. _________________	9. _________________
4. _________________	10. _________________
5. _________________	11. _________________
6. _________________	12. _________________

Vocabulary Activity

The following word search puzzle contains terms that are found in this chapter. Use the word list below to locate the hidden words in the grid.

```
C Q D R L R P R P I S O W T S U K U Z U
J F R K E Y O E Y B R A P D T D T P Y Y
R I B P Z S B B A F H U L C G O Y Q Q R
G K M Q B H I Z G V P P M E X L Y B O O
S G X P Y B G D E R Y X Y R Z G J G P S
Z H F R A I L N E S S K Q T B Q P E W B
Q F A H N I C B R N A K Q H J L E N E V
W L R E S T R A I N T S M V P V Y F V J
S B V A C Y P M T D N S B S F E B N G H
M R B Y C Z U Y E M P A T H Y V H Y T G
N X I V F Y M C U N S T A B L E G H A X
R O N D O N T U I X T H I F C N K M O A
W A N D E R G U A R D S W N B K G P C V
B E E Q X Y R F G Z N W G W X W P J X U
A B O L J P Q H M L P I Q B B J S Y Y X
V D E B U D N W R W S E W S K J M S P N
P P V Q O T E K N A L Z O Z A N H K N Y
W J Z C M Z I W G K I G S H K V H D U Y
S M B U E H Y X O J X Z E Q H A U J I W
T B V F V G F F X M F I F P L J P M K L
```

1. empathy
2. frailness
3. impairments
4. residents

5. restraints
6. unstable
7. wander guards

Developing Vocabulary

Writing Practice

Beside each word below, write a complete sentence using the word. For each sentence, check for accuracy of content, spelling, and punctuation.

1. empathy ____

   ____

   ____

2. wanderguards _______________________________________

   ____

   ____

3. residents ____

   ____

   ____

4. unstable ____

   ____

   ____

5. restraints ____

   ____

   ____

6. frailness____

   ____

   ____

7. impairments____

   ____

   ____

8. wandering____

   ____

   ____

True or False

If the definition on the right corresponds to the word on the left, then check True, if the word and definition do not correspond, check False.

TRUE	FALSE	WORD
____	____	1. **Restraints:** unsteady as in one's ability to walk
____	____	2. **Frailness:** weakness or infirmity that places the individual at risk for falling
____	____	3. **Unstable:** devices once used to tie an individual to a chair or bed for protective measures
____	____	4. **Residents:** individuals who live in nursing homes or in long-term care facilities
____	____	5. **Wanderguards:** alarms that sound when exit doors to LTC facilities are opened by the cognitively impaired for their own protection.

Spell Correctly

In each of the sets of words below, one word is spelled correctly. Circle the correctly spelled word.

1.
   a. restrasnts
   b. ristraints
   c. restraents
   d. restraints

2.
   a. wandergaurds
   b. wandergdards
   c. wanderguards
   d. wanderguerds

3.
   a. empithy
   b. emputhy
   c. empethy
   d. empathy

4.
   a. residents
   b. risidents
   c. residants
   d. residonts

5.
   a. impairments
   b. impiirments
   c. impaorments
   d. impiarments

Practice Scenario(s)

After reading this chapter in the text, read the following scenario(s) and answer the questions following each of them.

Situation 1

Emma Sharp is a resident of one month of Grand Canyon Manor, the nursing home where you work. Emma was directly discharged from the hospital as a permanent placement to your facility. There is no chance of her return to her small apartment. She came with no clothes or personal belongings other than the empty purse she refuses to surrender from her sight even when she is being transferred to the Century tub. Emma refuses to let anyone near her and has bitten several staff and residents who have come "too close." In the month at Grand Canyon Manor, she has tried to escape from the building numerous times. She has had no visitors since her arrival. Although alert the day of her arrival, she has been confused the last 3½ weeks.

Emma's roommate, Sarah Blum, approaches you about Emma. She wants her room changed because Emma keeps taking Sarah's clothes.

A team meeting is called regarding Emma Sharp. Her safety and the safety of others appears at risk because of the "attempted escapes" and biting. Someone brings up restraints.

1. What do you think is the cause of Emma's confusion?

    ____

    ____

    ____

2. Why does Emma refuse to let her empty purse out of her sight?

    ____

    ____

    ____

3. Why is Emma biting others?

    ____

    ____

    ____

4. What should you do when Sarah Blum reports that Emma is taking her clothes?

____

____

____

5. Based on the current guidelines and restraints policies, should restraints be considered as an option for Emma?

____

____

____

Situation 2

Mr. Lightfoot is a 96-year-old client with CHF and BPH. He is being seen for a UTI 2° indwelling catheter. Normally, he is alert and oriented. On today's visit, he seems lethargic and disoriented. As you prepare his meal in the kitchen, you smell something unusual. What should you do after smelling something unusual?

____

____

____

____

Situation 3

Mrs. Thomson is a 44-year-old paraplegic, who lives in a run-down neighborhood. Since the onset of her disability, she is unable to navigate the steps to the first floor where her kitchen is located. She has no family support and only one neighbor who checks in on her periodically. The phone in her bedroom upstairs is not by her bedside. The room is cluttered with outdated medications, newspapers, trash, leftover food, and dirty dishes. Twice the client has fallen and resorted to pulling herself across the floor to the window to yell for help. List

the unsafe conditions that are present in this situation; how would
you address or resolve each one of these conditions?

____

____

____

____

Situation 4

Mr. Wall is a 44-year-old truck driver and father of three children. He
had a CABG and was treated post-op in ICU for 36 hours. This
morning you assist the nurse in his transfer assessment and orientation
to your surgical unit. You and the RN note that he seems hesitant to
discuss his discharge needs and family relationships. He asks, "Why
do you need to know about my home life? I'm a patient in the hospital, not in the home." The nurse explains that a comprehensive
assessment involves discharge planning and that it is important to
consider the patient's needs in the hospital and post discharge. He
then explains that he and his wife separated three weeks before his
surgery. He tells you and the nurse that he will need minimal assistance from nursing staff in the hospital or home because he states, "I
can take care of myself. What I really need is rest and relaxation." I'll
call you when I need you."

You assume that Mr. Wall will call you when he needs assistance and
that the nurse will direct you in assisting him with any specific care
needs. You recognize his need for privacy and space so you "avoid"
entering his room unless it is essential.

On your 2:00 P.M. rounds you look into Mr. Wall's room and see him
lying on the floor. You enter the room, and he tells you, "I passed
out when I was getting up to go to the bathroom. I didn't think this
would happen to me."

1. What safety issue was neglected in the interest of meeting Mr.
   Walls's request for privacy?

____

____

____

2. What instructions should you and the nurse have provided Mr. Wall to assure safety without infringement on privacy?

____

____

____

Chapter 25

Essential Procdures and Tasks

Chapter Review

Multiple Choice

1. Time management involves
   a. assessing before planning.
   b. checking time frequently.
   c. accomplishing tasks swiftly.
   d. washing hands consistently.

2. Which one of the following statements demonstrates the principle of time management when making a bed?
   a. Avoid shaking the sheets.
   b. Smooth wrinkles from sheets.
   c. Complete one side completely.
   d. Raise the bed to a working level.

3. Temperature measured in the ear is called
   a. rectal.
   b. axillary.
   c. aural.
   d. oral.

4. The average respiratory rate is ___________ breaths per minute.
   a. 8 to 12
   b. 12 to 20
   c. 20 to 30
   d. 16 to 30

5. Which artery is used when measuring pulse at the wrist?
   a. carotid
   b. femoral
   c. aorta
   d. radial

6. When palpating a patient's pulse, you should note the strength or
   a. rate.   c. volume.
   b. rhythm.   d. character.

7. Diastolic pressure measures the force of blood against the walls of
   a. an artery during the relaxation phase.
   b. a vein during the contraction phase.
   c. an artery during the contraction phase.
   d. a vein during the relaxation phase.

8. According to the nursing process, which step involves bathing the patient?
   a. assess   c. implement
   b. plan   d. evaluate

9. If your patient drank 500 ml. of water, how many cc of water should be recorded?
   a. 1500   c. 250
   b. 500   d. 20

10. The measurement of a patient's weight provides information about the status of all but
    a. renal.
    b. nutritional.
    c. cardiovascular.
    d. neurologic.

11. Your patient micturated 8 ounces which would be recorded as
    __________ cc.
    a. 460   c. 500
    b. 240   d. 220

12. What happens if wastes are not eliminated from the body?
    a. edema
    b. dehydration
    c. jaundice
    d. death

13. Of the 4 steps below, which would be the first step to prepare a patient for meals?
    a. offer the bedpan
    b. brush teeth
    c. clean bedside table
    d. check tray for accuracy

14. Which bed position is used to assist the patient with dyspnea?
    a. Fowler's
    b. prone
    c. supine
    d. Sims'

Identification Exercise

Label the figure below:

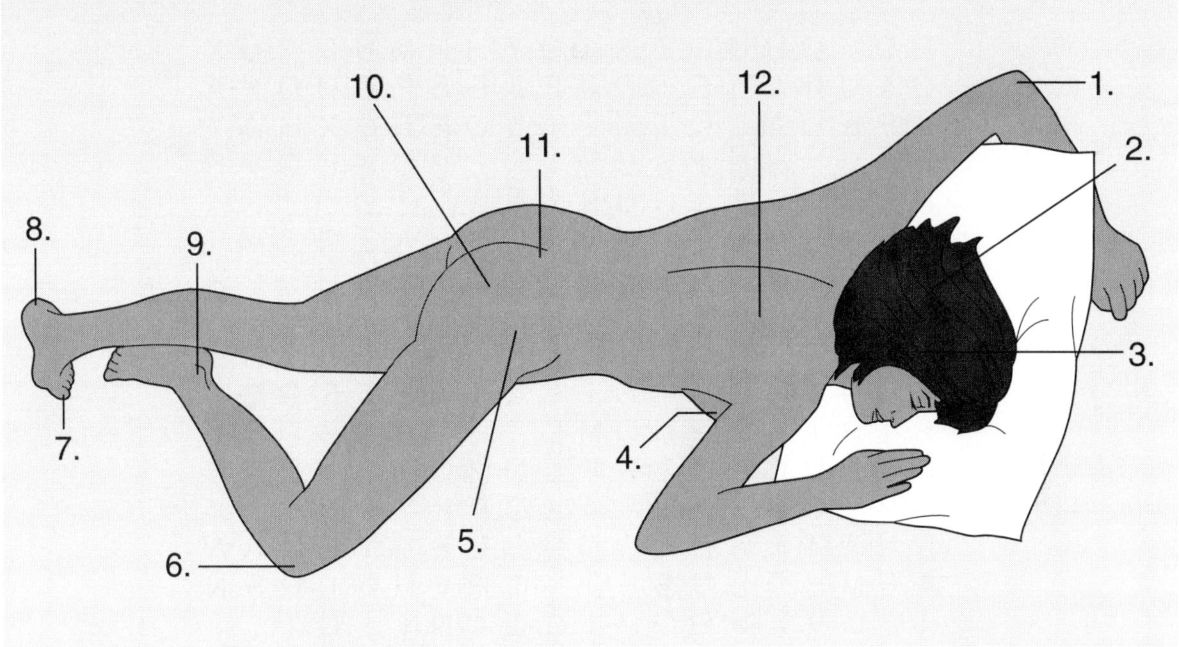

1._______________________	7._______________________
2._______________________	8._______________________
3._______________________	9._______________________
4._______________________	10._______________________
5._______________________	11._______________________
6._______________________	12._______________________

Vocabulary Activity

The following word search puzzle contains terms that are found in this chapter. Use the word list below to locate the hidden words in the grid.

```
B D Y D H U O Z A J O Y H U M N R C U X
O A U R A L E I U L E F E S F C M D Y A
J P E D A L Q T K E I L O P N Q X G W Y
F A B Y H H I S U P I N E U O K D D V P
H S W D E A T G U R Z H G T T D O Z R A
E E N E M A U A N V G R G U W Z O Z M T
V C D C E R F F M F O C M A T H E F X
C A P U L S E P S W E U R F L L G B U C
R R S B T L C J X G H N A D K V H D H U
E O U I G D Y Y D I C A T H E T E R C D
S T B T H E R M O M E T E R R N S P N V
P I H U C P N Z R P C O M O D G V P A C
I D Y S P H A G I A K O P K Y L R L L X
R N T J F G E C O C D S E E L Y H M W W
A E M B O L U S E T Y I R V H W L R R N
T I G V X V D Q M I Z Q A N I I D T Y I
I N C I S A L X P O P I T L F A F T I O
O G P V L K D R Y N J C U C V D J W K O
N P X A U Z Z M E R C U R Y R D T G S P
S P H Y G M O M A N O M E T E R T N W S
```

1. alignment	14. mercury
2. aural	15. pedal
3. carotid	16. pulse
4. catheter	17. radial
5. crutches	18. respirations
6. decubitus	19. sphygmomanometer
7. dysphagia	20. sputum
8. eggcrate	21. supine
9. embolus	22. temperature
10. enema	23. thermometer
11. impaction	24. turgor
12. incisal	25. walker
13. lingual	

Developing Vocabulary

Writing Practice

Beside each word below, write a complete sentence using the word. For each sentence, check for accuracy of content, spelling, and punctuation.

1. decubitus ___________________________________

____

____

2. respirations _________________________________

____

____

3. enema ______________________________________

____

____

4. catheter ____________________________________

____

____

5. aural _______________________________________

____

____

6. mercury _____________________________________

____

____

7. supine ______________________________________

____

____

8. sputum ______________________________________

____

____

True or False

If the definition on the right corresponds to the word on the left, then check True, if the word and definition do not correspond, check False.

TRUE   FALSE   WORD

____   ____   1. **Turgor:** elasticity of the skin

____   ____   2. **Pulse:** the wave of oxygenated blood sent through the arteries with each heart beat

____   ____   3. **Incisal:** traveling blood clot

____   ____   4. **Alignment:** refers to the correct positioning and joint support of the patient's spine and extremities

____   ____   5. **Impaction:** hardened stools trapped in the lower colon

Spell Correctly

In each of the sets of words below, one word is spelled correctly. Circle the correctly spelled word.

1.   a. sphygmomanumeter   c. sphygmomnaometer
        b. sphygmomanometir   d. sphygmomanometer

2.   a. emboles   c. embolas
        b. embolus   d. emmolus

3.   a. thermomiter   c. thermometer
        b. thremometer   d. thermometar

4.   a. caretid   c. carutid
        b. carotid   d. carosid

5.   a. dysphagea   c. dssphagia
        b. dysphhgia   d. dysphagia

Practice Scenario(s)

After reading this chapter in the text, read the following scenario(s) and answer the questions following each of them.

Situation 1

Mrs. Kief is a 90-year-old patient who has diabetes mellitus and is blind. She recently had a left radical mastectomy. You are required to check her blood pressure twice this shift. In assessing and planning personal care for this patient, what factors should be considered?

____

____

____

____

Situation 2

Mr. Tobar is a 75-year-old resident on the dementia unit of the nursing home where you work. He is a new resident in your assignment. He has just been transferred from the hospital after being treated with C. diff. This is the information that you are given in morning report: Incontinent of urine and stool; Temperature of 101 degrees Fahrenheit; VS at 9 a.m.; daily weight this a.m.; recreation activity at 9 a.m.; bath in the Century tub.

1. What plan should be made for Mr. Tobar's morning care?

____

____

____

2. What should you assess in this situation?

____

____

____

Situation 3

Mr. Taglieb is a resident who suffers from dementia and is frequently confused and agitated. The nurse instructs you to take his tempeature STAT. What should you assess and plan in this situation?

____

____

____

____

Situation 4

You are working the evening shift on a surgical patient care unit. Your assignment includes the following tasks, which must be completed for a fresh post-op patient:

1. Using the principle of time management, organize and priortize the tasks listed: Instruct patient on use of incentive spirometer; STAT vital signs; change gown and bottom sheet (patient has been bleeding); 12-lead ECG; venous blood sample for CBC and Chem 7.

____

____

____

2. Rate the tasks from 1 to 5 (1 is most important, and 5 is least important.)

____

____

____

C h a p t e r   2 6

Advanced or Expanded Procedures and Tasks

Chapter Review

Multiple Choice

1. Straight urinary catheterization procedure may be performed to
   a. obtain a sterile specimen.
   b. administer 24° irrigation.
   c. drain urine continuously.
   d. monitor I&O post-operative.

2. Urinary bladder catheterization is a __________ procedure.
   a. clean
   b. aseptic
   c. sterile
   d. surgical

3. When inserting a Foley in a male patient, insert the tube __________ inches into the urethra.
   a. 2 to 3
   b. 1 to 2
   c. 4 to 5
   d. 6 to 7

4. An NG tube is ordered for all except
   a. temporary feeding method.
   b. stomach contents drainage.
   c. stomach decompression.
   d. endoscopic procedures.

5. PEG tube feedings must be done with the patient in a __________ position.
   a. Fowler's
   b. Sims'
   c. prone
   d. supine

6. Before administering a PEG tube feeding, you must
   a. measure output.
   b. measure residual.
   c. take vital signs.
   d. lower the bed.

7. A test that you might perform to measure and record the electrical activity of the heart is an
   a. ERG.   c. EEG.
   b. ECG.   d. EMG.

8. When applying the precordial leads for an electrocardiogram, V_3 is placed
   a. on the right sternal border.
   b. on the 5th intercostal space mid-axilla.
   c. midway between V_2 and V_4.
   d. parallel to V_1

9. If a patient has a tremor of the extremities, the limb leads should be placed close to the trunk to reduce the
   a. presence of artifact.
   b. patient from shaking.
   c. presence of 60 cycle.
   d. baseline from wandering.

10. A patient with a normal functioning sigmoid colostomy would probably evacuate what type of excreta?
    a. liquid green   c. pale yellow
    b. pasty dark   d. formed brown

11. The type of dressing that acts as a second skin is
    a. Tegaderm.   c. wet-to-dry.
    b. duoderm.   d. saline.

12. Of the tubes of blood ordered to be drawn, which would be first?
    a. lavender   c. gray
    b. green   d. blue

13. A hematoma resulting from the phlebotomy procedure is caused by
    a. thrombosed veins.
    b. venous inflammation.
    c. blood leakage.
    d. trauma phlebitis.

14. An oximetry value that has increased greater than _________ percent should be reported.
    a. 5   c. 15
    b. 10   d. 20

Vocabulary Activity

The following word search puzzle contains terms that are found in this chapter. Use the word list below to locate the hidden words in the grid.

```
C A T H E T E R I Z A T I O N M K R F M
N S T C K X F R E N C H A O C A L B W P
X P J S Z X P H L E B O T O M Y I R Y A
P I T E G A D E R M B O L U S X D F Q M
Y R J I O L I V C D V A Y O X I T S L L
A A O W I L E O S T O M Y Z S A V Y M O
N T P E R C U S S I O N V B Y T V D Z P
K E Q R J T D U O D E R M C W K O U S C
E K Y B P R E C O R D I A L Y M N M T O
U R I N O M E T E R E V H T Y P H Q Y D
R S C K E V Z I O C A S M X E C Z Z L R
O X I S E N S O R K K M I Q M E I M U V
S H V S L I O N U E O H Y D I R Z J S X
T K U B Y H B I P P V R T J U M V Y U G
O U K M U H E N K S X V V W G A J V X X
M T G H Q W L G C H Y X C K F O L E Y V
Y R S P N C A C W X C Z O J U W G O M T
C F B F A Z M B M T C V Y X S P S G O X
J G T J Q A T V L T S Q X A Z O X Z L P
R W M T Z B X Q J T I W K T C B S G A U
```

1. aspirate	11. percussion
2. bolus	12. phlebotomy
3. catheterization	13. precordial
4. colostomy	14. residual
5. duoderm	15. stylus
6. expectorate	16. suctioning
7. foley	17. tegaderm
8. french	18. urinometer
9. ileostomy	19. urostomy
10. oxisensor	20. yankeur

Developing Vocabulary

Writing Practice

Beside each word below, write a complete sentence using the word. For each sentence, check for accuracy of content, spelling, and punctuation.

1. yankeur ____

____

____

2. urostomy ____

____

____

3. tegaderm ____

____

____

4. urinometer ____

____

____

5. colostomy ____

____

____

6. french gauge ____

____

____

7. percussion ____

____

____

8. aspirate ____

____

____

True or False

If the definition on the right corresponds to the word on the left, then check True, if the word and definition do not correspond, check False.

TRUE	FALSE	WORD
____	____	1. **Expectorate:** a respiratory care procedure in which cupped hands are tapped over the thoracic area to dislodge mucus
____	____	2. **Precordial:** synonym for the six chest or V leads leading from the central cable of the ECG machine
____	____	3. **Suctioning:** the process of withdrawing secretions of fluids from an airway with a catheter
____	____	4. **Bolus:** a concentrated mass administered rapidly, as in medicine
____	____	5. **Percussion:** puncturing a vein to obtain a venous blood sample for lab analysis

Spell Correctly

In each of the sets of words below, one word is spelled correctly. Circle the correctly spelled word.

1.   a. stylus   c. stylas
         b. stilus   d. styles

2.   a. oxisensor   c. oxusensor
         b. oxixensor   d. oxisensir

3.   a. phlebotomy   c. phlebetomy
         b. phlabotomy   d. phlebotumy

4.   a. ileostomy   c. ilaostomy
         b. iliostomy   d. ileomtomy

5.   a. expoctorate   c. expectorate
         b. expectarate   d. expecoorate

Practice Scenario(s)

After reading this chapter in the text, read the following scenario(s) and answer the questions following each of them.

Situation 1

Mr. Simmons has a PEG tube through which he receives bolus feedings. You withdraw 180 cc of residual stomach contents.

1. What should you assess before you begin the tube feeding?

   ____

   ____

   ____

2. What is your plan for withdrawing 180 cc of residual stomach contents?

   ____

   ____

   ____

Situation 2

Mrs. Marks has four lab studies ordered this morning. She is a patient who receives outpatient dialysis treatments, and she has an AV shunt in her left arm.

1. What should you include in the pre-procedure assessment?

   ____

   ____

   ____

2. What do you need to plan?

   ____

   ____

   ____

Situation 3

Mr. Haab is a 79-year-old male who has COPD. He was admitted yeaterday in CHF, and he has pneumonia. You are assigned to perform an ECG STAT because of chest pain. You must also perform a pulse OX and chest percussion, cough, and deep breathe. The ECG has a significant amount of artifact. You complete the pulse OX, and it is 89. Pulse OX was last measured two hours ago, and it was 98. During chest PT, Mr. Haab begins to cough uncontrollably.

1. What task will you perform first, and why?

   ____

   ____

   ____

2. What do you plan to do regarding the ECG results?

   ____

   ____

   ____

3. What do you do regarding the pulse OX results?

   ____

   ____

   ____

4. What do you do regarding Mr. Haab's uncontrollable cough during chest PT?

   ____

   ____

   ____

Situation 4

Mr. Glover has been diagnosed with Crohn's disease. Yesterday, he arrived on your unit post-op after having an ileostomy. You are assigned to perform A.M. care for this patient. In report, you are given the following information: assist with ADLs; VS q.4h; clear liquid diet; OOB to chair with assistance; empty ostomy appliance prn.

1. How do you plan to proceed with his care this morning?

____

____

____

C h a p t e r   2 7

Clinical and Environmental Emergencies

Chapter Review

Multiple Choice

1. The type of seizure that produces tonic-clonic muscle contractions is
   a. petit mal.
   b. Jacksonian.
   c. grand mal.
   d. temporal lobe.

2. When a patient has a grand mal seizure, you should not
   a. protect the limbs from injury.
   b. loosen restrictive clothing.
   c. use a padded tongue blade.
   d. move furniture out of the way.

3. The "A" of the ABC's of CPR stands for
   a. artery.
   b. airway.
   c. apply.
   d. alternate.

4. When do you check for a pulse when performing CPR?
   a. after opening the airway
   b. after giving two (2) successful breaths
   c. after starting chest compressions
   d. before activating the E.M.S.

5. When performing CPR if the first breath is unsuccessful, you should
   a. reestablish the airway.
   b. give five (5) abdominal thrusts.
   c. palpate the carotid pulse.
   d. activate the E.M.S.

6. A patient in shock should be placed in the __________ position.
   a. Fowler's
   b. Sims'
   c. Trendelenburg
   d. recumbent

7. Before attempting the Heimlich maneuver on a possible choking victim, you should
   a. activate the E.M.S. and perform the Heimlich.
   b. seat the patient and establish an airway.
   c. ask the patient if he is choking and can speak.
   d. give five (5) back blows and evaluate.

8. The "R" in R.A.C.E. stands for
   a. run.
   b. rescue.
   c. race.
   d. reflect.

9. After removing persons from the immediate area of a fire, you should
   a. evacuate the building.
   b. extinguish the fire.
   c. contain the smoke.
   d. sound the alarm.

10. Electrical safety precautions include all except
    a. checking outlets before use.
    b. reporting frayed wires.
    c. inspecting electrical devices.
    d. using extension cords.

11. Electrical safety is the responsibility of the
    a. supervising nurse.
    b. facility staff.
    c. house electricians.
    d. biomedical engineers.

12. Acids, alcohol products, correction fluid, and mercury are examples of
    a. M.S.D.S.
    b. cleaning agents.
    c. HAZMATS.
    d. corrosive agents.

13. Key words that identify health hazards on an MSDS include all but
    a. irritant.
    b. pathogen.
    c. toxin.
    d. carcinogen.

14. In working with hazardous material, your role as a CCA is to
    a. update MSDS log monthly.
    b. use the correct protective equipment.
    c. treat injuries resulting from HAZMATS.
    d. lock all HAZMATS in clean utility room.

Vocabulary Activity

The following crossword puzzle contains terms that are found in this chapter. Use the clues below to complete the puzzle.

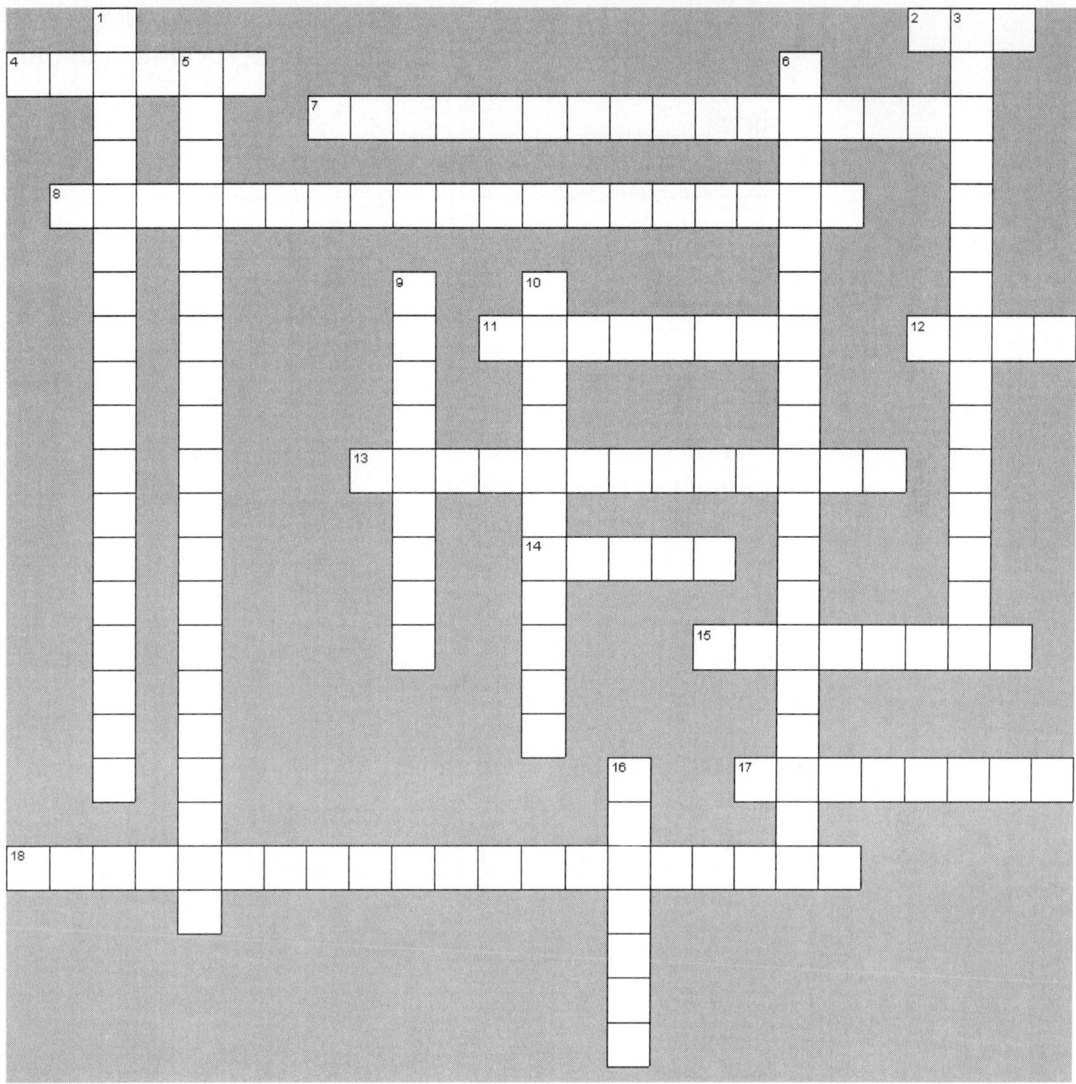

ACROSS

2. temporary method of providing breaths and chest compressions to victims of cardiac arrest
4. injury to the body
7. techniques for removing an airway obstruction from a choking victim
8. seizures varied in appearance; result of temporal lobe malfunction
11. small seizures
12. product information provided by manufacturer of hazardous materials
13. heart ceases to beat
14. warning signal that the body is in grave danger
15. a disorder in which the primary symptom is seizure
17. "full blown" seizure
18. epilepsy in which seizures occur that result from temporal lobe malfunction

DOWN

1. seizures that involve one side of the body
3. seizures in which part of the cerebrum is involved
5. cardiac tissue death caused by blockage of the coronary arteries
6. seizures in which all of the cerebrum is involved
9. blood, body fluid, or item contaminated with body fluids
10. shock caused by massive infections and adverse reaction to medications
16. condition of electrical disturbances in the brain

Developing Vocabulary

Writing Practice

Beside each word below, write a complete sentence using the word. For each sentence, check for accuracy of content, spelling, and punctuation.

1. shock

2. cardiac arrest

3. temporal lobe epilepsy

4. psychomotor seizures

5. CPR

6. biohazard

7. trauma

8. MSDS

True or False

If the definition on the right corresponds to the word on the left, then check True, if the word and definition do not correspond, check False.

TRUE	FALSE	WORD
____	____	1. **Jacksonian seizures:** seizures that involve one side of the body
____	____	2. **Septic shock:** epilepsy in which seizures occur that result from temporal lobe malfunction
____	____	3. **Cardiac arrest:** the heart ceases to beat
____	____	4. **Generalized seizures:** those seizures in which part of the cerebrum is involved
____	____	5. **Trauma:** shock caused by massive infections and adverse reaction to medications

Spell Correctly

In each of the sets of words below, one word is spelled correctly. Circle the correctly spelled word.

1. a. infurction   c. infarction
   b. infarctoin   d. infarcsion

2. a. myocardial   c. myocardail
   b. myocardeal   d. mdocardial

3. a. seisure   c. seizzre
   b. siezure   d. seizure

4. a. mnaeuver   c. maneuver
   b. meneuver   d. manouver

5. a. epilepsy   c. epulepsy
   b. epilapsy   d. epelepsy

Practice Scenario(s)

After reading this chapter in the text, read the following scenario(s) and answer the questions following each of them.

Situation 1

Mr. Cohn, an 88-year-old homebound client, is being followed post-MI. Following A.M. care, Mr. Cohn c/o of dizziness and, in seconds, loses consciousness. Upon assessment of Mr. Cohn, you observe that he is not breathing. You are able to give Mr. Cohn two effective breaths. Mr. Cohn has no carotid pulse. When the ambulance arrives at 9:40, you say that the patient became unconscious after A.M. care, which was at 9:31. You initiated CPR at 9:33 A.M.

1. What is your first response when Mr. Cohn loses consciousness?

____

____

____

2. When you discover that Mr. Cohn is not breathing, what is your next step?

____

____

____

3. How did you determine the absence of breathing?

____

____

____

4. What is your next step after you give Mr. Cohn two effective breaths?

____

____

____

5. What intervention is next when you discover that Mr. Cohn has no carotid pulse?

____

____

____

6. From what emergency condition did the patient suffer?

____

____

____

7. Was CPR initiated before brain damage occurs?

____

____

____

Situation 2

John Rocket is your assigned patient on the neurology service. He has a history of petit mal seizures. Recently, he has had many petit mal seizures. You are transferring him into a chair to eat his lunch and he says to you, "I smell bread baking." He then lets out a cry and begins to fall to the floor.

1. What do you do?

____

____

____

Then, John begins to have jerking motions of his arms and legs; his head is in danger of banging the floor. He has frothy saliva coming from his mouth and his lips are turning blue.

2. What actions will you take?

____

____

____

The nurse arrives and you describe the details of the event. The nurse asks if there was any warning sign or aura.

1. Were there any warning signs or aura?

____

____

____

The nurse asks what you think just occurred. The nurse and you return John to bed and find that he has been incontinent of urine. He says he has a headache and wants to sleep.

2. What interventions will you take now?

____

____

____

Situation 3

Mrs. Denlinger is a 68-year-old who is being followed at home following a compression fracture of L_5 secondary to osteoporosis. She also suffers from COPD. This morning while she is eating her breakfast, she begins to cough. Her face is bright red and she is struggling.

1. What should you do?

____

____

____

Mrs. Denlinger coughs until she is blue and no longer is coughing. She is making no sounds at all.

2. What is your next strategy?

____

____

____

3. From what type of airway obstruction is Mrs. Denlinger suffering?

____

____

____

Mrs. Denlinger passes out onto the floor of the kitchen. She does not appear to be breathing.

4. What is your next plan of action?

____

____

____

Situation 4

Henry Prezuski is a resident in the CRR. He is found smoking in his bedroom and the resident counselor tells him to put out the cigarette. He should smoke in the designated area on the ground floor of the house. An hour later you smell smoke coming from upstairs. Other residents are sleeping in their bedrooms. You find that Mr. Prezuski's room is in flames and smoke is coming into the hallway. You last saw Mr. P. in the kitchen eating a sandwich.

1. What is your first action?

____

____

____

2. What word should you call to mind immediately to respond?

____

____

____

Situation 5

While you are changing bed linens, you are stuck with a needle that was in the linens. To what risk have you been exposed and what should you do?

____

____

____

____

Glossary

24-hour urine specimen Collection of a patient's urine over a 24-hour period; used for testing purposes (25)

Escherichia coli (E. coli) Colon bacillus; short, plump, gram-negative, nonspore-forming motile bacilli almost constantly present in the alimentary canal of humans and other animals (23)

abduction Act of moving a part away from the midline of the body (9)

absorption The process by which broken down nutrients pass into the bloodstream through capillaries into the small intestine to be utilized as necessary (18)

absorption The process of transferring nutrient molecules into the circulating blood so they can be distributed and used by the cells of the body (13)

acceptance One of the five stages of death and dying in which a person comes to grips with the diagnosis, the treatment, the pain and the truth, and the living of each moment for all that it holds (20)

ACE Bandage Trade name for an elastic bandage made of woven material (25)

acne An inflammatory disease of the sebaceous glands (7)

acoustic nerve Nerve which transmits the impulses received in the hearing receptors to the temporal lobe for interpretation of the sounds heard (10)

acromegaly Abnormal enlargement of the extremities, especially the jaws, hands, and feet (16)

active assist Participation of the patient with the caregiver in performing the procedure (25)

active range-of-motion exercises Exercises performed by the patient unassisted (25)

activities of daily living (ADLs) Daily routine tasks such as eating, dressing, and bathing (5)

acute gastritis Inflammation of the mucous membrane of the stomach that can be related to dietary intake of irritating food, medications, alcohol, or can be a sign of infection of the GI system (13)

Addison's disease Results from deficient secretion of the cortisol hormones from the adrenal cortex (16)

adduction Act of moving a part toward the midline of the body (9)

adipose capsule A fatty protection around the kidneys, which also cushions them (14)

adrenal glands Glands located on top of the kidneys (16)

adrenaline One of the neurochemicals that is also a hormone; stimulates or accelerates reactions; adrenaline is also called epinephrine (10)

adrenocorticotrophic hormone (ACTH) Pituitary hormone that stimulates the cortex of the adrenals to produce adrenal cortical hormones (16)

advanced directive A legally valid written or oral statement that designates an individual's treatment decisions and a surrogate decision maker (20)

agnostic One who holds the view that any ultimate reality is unknown and probably unknowable (19)

Airborne isolation precautions Precautions designed to reduce the transmission of certain diseases, e.g. tuberculosis, measles, chicken pox (23)

airborne precautions Isolation criteria for all suspected cases of communicable diseases by transmission through air (12)

albumin Blood protein (11)

aldosterone Mineralcorticoid that helps to regulate the concentration of minerals in the body (16)

aldosterone Salt-retaining hormone (14)

alimentary canal The digestive tube from the mouth to the anus (13)

alpha cells Cells in the islet of Langerhans that produce the hormone glucagon (16)

alveolus Air cell found in clusters at the endings of the bronchioles of the lungs; the site of O_2 and CO_2 exchange (12)

Alzheimer's disease   The degeneration of neurons and the accumulation of tangles and plaques of the neurons in the forebrain in which there is a great loss of neurons; the individual may demonstrate agitated behavior, paranoid thinking, depression, euphoria, or lack of recognition of daily events and people (21)

ambivalence   Inability to make a decision because both sides of the situation seem equal (22)

ambulatory care services   Care services for which an individual can "walk in"; services in which persons are treated in the community by primary doctors in private practice, in group practices that are not associated with a hospital or group, or in private practices that are associated with a hospital or health maintenance organization (2)

ambulatory   The ability to ambulate or walk (2)

American Diabetes Association (ADA)   Association that establishes guidelines used to prescribe the diabetic diet (16)

amino acids   The substances created when proteins are broken down; there are 22 amino acids, nine of which are essential (18)

ammonia   Organic waste found in urine (14)

anatomy   The study of the structure of an organism (6)

androgens   Male sex hormones (16)

anemia   Disorder in which hemoglobin, the oxygen carrying component of the blood, is low (11)

aneroid sphygmomanometer   Type of blood pressure apparatus that uses a dial with a needle gauge (25)

aneurysms   Localized dilation of a blood vessel wall (11)

anger   One of the five stages of death and dying in which a person expresses resentment of reality manifested physically by aggressive behavior or verbally with caustic remarks; it can be covert or overt (20)

angina pectoris   Paroxysmal chest pain caused by myocardial anoxia; warning signal of a decrease of oxygen supply to the heart muscle (11)

angina   Spasmodic, cramp-like, choking sensation (11)

anterior (ventral)   Front side of the body or structure (6)

anterior lobe   One of the two portions of the pituitary gland (16)

antibodies   Immunoglobulin essential to the immune system (11)

antidiuretic hormone (ADH)   Hormone produced by the posterior pituitary that stimulates the tubules of the kidneys to reabsorb water; "water-retaining hormone" (16)

antidiuretic hormone (ADH)   Water-retaining hormone (14)

antiembolism stockings   Stockings worn by patients to prevent post-operative circulatory complications, such as traveling blood clots (Also called therapeutic stockings or hose; surgical stockings or hose; TED hose or stockings; JOBST hose or stockings.) (25)

antigens   Substance, usually proteins, that causes the formation of an antibody (11)

antiprostaglandin anti-inflammatory   Medication used to reduce the effects of prostaglandin or tissue hormones during menstruation (15)

antisocial personality disorder   Disorder that results in irresponsible behavior and the inability to conform to social norms (21)

anuria   Absence of urine (14)

anus   Sphincter muscle with an inner involuntary muscle and an outer voluntary muscle that opens for defecation of solid waste (13)

anxiety disorders   Disorders that stem from distorted perception of events and fall into the categories of general anxiety, panic disorders, phobias, and dissociative disorders (21)

anxiety   Generalized feelings of fear and apprehension (22)

aorta   Largest artery in the body (11)

apnea   "Without breathing"; breathing has stopped (12)

appendicitis   Inflammation of the blind pouch in the right lower quadrant of the abdominol pelvic cavity (13)

appendicular   One of the two subdivisions of the skeletal system; it includes the shoulder girdle, arms, hands, hips, legs, and feet (8)

appendix   A small blind process projecting from the end of the cecum in the right lower quadrant (13)

areola   Pigmented circular area around the nipple of the breast (15)

arrectores pilorum   The muscle fibers that help to keep heat in the body; literally, "erectors of hair" (7)

arrhythmias   Any deviations from the normal heartbeat pattern (11)

arterioles   Small arteries (11)

artery   Large blood vessel that carries blood away from the heart (11)

articulation   The union of two or more bones (8)

ascending colon   Part of the colon that travels up the right side of the abdominal cavity (13)

asepsis   Being free from infection (23)

aseptic technique   Maintaining cleanliness and eliminating or preventing contamination (23)

aspirate To withdraw by force, as in the removal of undigested nutritional supplement and gastric juices remaining during tube feeding (26)

aspiration pneumonia Occurs when a large amount of residual in the stomach plus an added new feeding causes backflow of stomach contents into the esophagus and causes vomiting with backflow into the lungs (26)

aspiration pneumonia Pneumonia, or inflammation of the lungs, caused by aspiration of fluids such as stomach contents that are breathed in during vomiting (12)

aspiration Act of breathing vomitus or an object into the lungs; occurs when the trachea is blocked by food or any object, and air cannot enter the lungs (12)

assessing Step in the nursing process in which the nurse identifies a problem and decides what needs to be done to solve it (17)

assimilation The sum of physical and chemical changes and all energy and material transformations that take place in the body (18)

assistance with a tub bath or shower Providing help with towels and supplies, preparing the water, supervising, and assisting (25)

asthma Condition caused by intermittent obstruction of the bronchial tubes (12)

atelectasis Collapsing of a lung (12)

atrioventricular (AV) node An area of special cardiac tissue that receives and transmits cardiac signal as part of the heart's conduction system (11)

atrophy Muscle wasting (9)

attorney-in-fact A surrogate decision maker who makes treatment decisions for the individual when the patient is unable to make those decisions personally (20)

aural temperature Method of measuring body temperature by the external ear (25)

auscultation Process of listening to breathing sounds with a stethoscope (12)

autoclave Piece of equipment used to sterilize articles by way of steam under pressure and/or dry heat (23)

autonomic nervous system (ANS) Subsystem of the nervous system, which is involved with involuntary and automatic control of the glands and organs of the entire body (10)

autonomy Means to be self-directed and to do for oneself (19)

avoidant personality disorder Disorder that manifests as general fear, fear of negative evaluation, and great social discomfort (21)

axial One of the two subdivisions of the skeletal system; it includes the bones of the cranium, face, spinal column, and chest (8)

axon One of the three main parts to a neuron, which extends from the cell body and conducts messages away from the cell body (10)

bargaining One of the five stages of death and dying in which a person responds to impending death by making promises or deals with God (20)

Bartholin's gland Exocrine glands that lie lateral to the vaginal opening that secrete a lubricating fluid (15)

basal metabolic rate (BMR) Resting rate of a person's metabolism when no voluntary work is being performed (18)

base of support The way which the body moves and maintains balance (23)

baselining Analyzing a behavior that requires modification (22)

bathing Personal hygiene that includes the entire body (25)

bedsores Synonym for decubitus; caused by prolonged pressure (25)

behavior modification A treatment technique that helps to reduce the occurrence of undesirable or unwanted behavior (22)

behavior The actions or responses that one produces in reaction to a given stimulus (22)

beneficence The assumption that the professional training and judgment of health care professionals will direct them to act in the best interest of the patient because they know what is good for the patient (17)

benign Noncancerous (10)

beta cells Cells in the islet of Langerhans that produce the hormone insulin (16)

bicuspid Having two cusps or points (11)

bile A green-yellow alkaline liquid (produced by the liver and stored in the gallbladder) that helps to neutralize acid, emulsify fats, and remove toxins from the liver (13)

biohazard Any blood product, body fluid, or item contaminated with blood or body fluids that may be a "life hazard" (27)

bipolar mood disorder Disorder that is characterized by episodes of mania and depression (21)

bladder Muscular reservoir for urine storage from the kidneys (14)

blood pressure Measurement of the force exerted by the blood against the arterial walls when the heart contracts and relaxes (25)

blood pressure The force against the artery walls as the heart contracts and relaxes (11)

body alignment   Refers to the correct positioning and joint support of the patient's head, spine, and extremities (25)

body mechanisms   Principle used to describe the way a body moves (23)

body system   Synonym for system (6)

body temperature   Average temperature of 98.6 (25)

bolus method   A method of tube feeding that involves three or four feedings during a 24-hour period (26)

bone spurs   Growths of excess bone located along the joint edges of the bones (8)

booting up the system   The process of turning on the computer (3)

borderline personality disorder   Disorder that is characterized by unstable moods, self-image, and inconsistent interpersonal relationships (21)

Bowman's capsule   Kidney tissue that surrounds the glomerulus (14)

bradycardia   Heart rate less than 60 beats per minute (11)

brain stem   One of the major parts of the brain consisting of the medulla oblongata, pons, and midbrain; the portion of the brain that connects to the spinal cord (10)

breasts   Mammary glands that produce and release milk to nourish an infant child (15)

bronchi   Organs of the respiratory system that act as passageways that support air cells (12)

bronchioles   Bronchial passageways that support clusters of air cells throughout the entire surface of the lungs (12)

buccal cavity   The mouth; a cavity formed by the jaw bones and the palate (13)

buccal   Surface of the tooth nearest the cheek (25)

bulbourethral glands   One of the glands that produce seminal fluid (15)

calcitonin   Hormone involved in the regulation of blood calcium levels (16)

calcium   A mineral that is stored by the bones of the skeletal system and serves to give them strength and stability of shape (8)

calcium   Mineral salt necessary for bone growth and metabolism (14)

cancellous   Bone tissue that is spongy and porous (8)

capillaries   Thin-walled tiny blood vessels joining arterioles and venules (11)

carbohydrates   Made of carbon, hydrogen, and oxygen, they come from such foods as grains, cereals, legumes, nuts, vegetables, and fruits (18)

cardiac arrest   The heart ceases to beat (27)

cardiac catheterization   Diagnostic surgical procedure in which a catheter is passed through the femoral artery into the heart and dye is introduced to visualize the coronary arteries (11)

cardiomegaly   Abnormally enlarged heart (11)

cardiovascular (CV)   Pertaining to the heart and the blood vessels (11)

carotid pulse   Pulse assessed to determine whether the heart is pumping blood to the brain (25)

cartilage   Tough connective tissue that covers the ends of bones and acts like a rubber cushion, softening the shock of movement (8)

catatonia   Absence of body movements (21)

catatonic schizophrenia   A psychotic disorder dominated by any of the following: catatonic stupor or mutism; catatonic negativism; catatonic rigidity; catatonic excitement; catatonic posturing (21)

catheterization kit   A prepackaged collection of supplies needed for inserting a catheter using a sterile technique (26)

catheterization   The insertion of a sterile tube into the urinary bladder (26)

catheters   Flexible tubes used to drain fluids from the body (25)

causative agent   The particular microbe that causes a disease (23)

CD-ROM drive   The port on a computer where CDs arc inserted, just like a CD player (3)

cell body   One of the three main parts to a neuron, which contains the nucleus of the neuron and is the brain of a nerve cell; it changes the nature and direction of the signals that pass through it (10)

cell membrane   Thin layer of cells that act as a boundary between the cell contents and the outside environment (6)

cell   Unit of structure of all organisms (6)

Centers of Disease Control (CDC)   Division of the U.S. Public Health Service in Atlanta, Georgia; for investigation and control of various diseases (23)

central nervous system (CNS)   One of the two main divisions of the nervous system, which is composed of the brain and the spinal cord. It is located in the center of the body and is the center for processing all nervous activity (10)

central processing unit (CPU)   The computer's brain (3)

central venous pressure   Blood pressure in the large veins of the body (11)

centrifuge   Device for separating components of liquid, as in blood products (11)

cerebellum Located under the occipital lobe, this brain structure is involved in the production of normal body movements (10)

cerebral vascular accident (CVA) Synonym for a stroke; caused by hemorrhage or blood clots that form in a blood vessel in the brain or clots that travel to the brain (10)

cerebrum Largest section of the human brain, which makes us think, feel, reason, imagine, create, see, hear, feel, smell, and taste (10)

certificate A document (not a license) that is issued by a representative organization or association to individuals who have passed the association's certification examination; this adds credibility to the title and generally tells employers that these individuals have the minimum competence expected by the association (3)

certified nurse practitioner A registered nurse who has a master's degree in a particular field of nursing (2)

cervix Neck that opens to the vagina from the uterus (15)

chaining The process of teaching a task step-by-step and linking each step together like the links of a chain (22)

chemical digestion Digestion that involves the work that stomach acid, bile, and a variety of enzymes have on changing mechanically digested food into absorbable molecules of nutrient substances (13)

Cheyne-Stokes Respirations observed when someone is near death (12)

chloride Negative electrolyte (14)

cholesterol Fatlike substance that circulates in the blood as lipoproteins (18)

choroid Second continuous layer of the eyeball (10)

chromosomes One of the bodies in the cell nucleus that carries genes (6)

chronic bronchitis Chronic obstructive pulmonary disease (12)

chronic gastritis Inflammation of the mucous membrane of the stomach that changes the mucous lining of the stomach (13)

chronic obstructive pulmonary disease (COPD) General term used to describe the diseases chronic bronchitis, asthma, and emphysema (12)

cilia Tiny hairlike structures that line the mucous membrane of the nose (12)

circumcision Surgical procedure used to remove the foreskin of the penis after birth (15)

classifieds The section of the newspaper that lists available jobs within the community; the medical section often holds the largest list of prospective jobs (4)

clients Outpatient, home care, day clinic consumers of health services (2)

clinical care associate (CCA) An individual who performs the tasks of the nursing assistant, an ECG technician, and a phlebotomist, and who also performs simple respiratory treatments (3)

clinical experiences Practical experience without pay in which certain skills are practiced; this can provide a great job lead (4)

clinitest/acetest tablet Reagent tablet that, when in contact with urine, tests for sugar or acetone content (25)

clitoris Small projection of erectile tissue with nerves and blood vessels (15)

closed bed Bed made after a patient is discharged (25)

cognitive disorder Disorder caused directly by a physical defect in the brain that impairs normal brain functions (21)

cold applications Therapeutic used to relieve pain and reduce swelling, reduce body temperature, control bleeding (25)

colitis Inflammation of the colon or large bowel (13)

collaboration Working/laboring together (17)

colostomy Created by opening the large intestine and forming a stoma (hole) of colon tissue on the surface of the abdomen (26)

colostomy Surgical procedures in which a portion or all of the colon is removed (13)

colostrum A thin, yellow liquid that provides an immense amount of immune protection in the first six months of an infant's life (18)

combining vowel A vowel that is used in the combination and hookup between prefixes, roots, and suffixes in word building (5)

commercially prepared (Fleet) enemas Disposable container with 4 to 6 ounces of solution usually hypertonic; used to stimulate peristalsis and eliminate stool (25)

commitment Dedication to the work of a team (17)

communication Complex process that involves verbal and nonverbal messages (17)

compact Bone tissue that is dense and strong (8)

competencies Accomplishments and learning of a life stage (19)

competent A term used to describe a person who is able to recognize, comprehend, and weigh the risks of alternative treatment options (20)

complete care Care given by the nurse when the patient cannot assist (25)

complete proteins Proteins containing all nine essential amino acids (18)

compound fracture   A broken bone when the bone protrudes through the skin (8)

compulsion   The action that is used to relieve the anxiety produced by an obsessive thought (22)

concave   One of the four normal curves of the spine; the cervical and lumbar areas are concave (curved inward) (8)

concussion   Temporary loss of consciousness as the result of a blow to the head (10)

cones   Specialized microscopic receptors in the eye that respond to light rays that enter the retina; they are sensitive to bright light and are important for good vision in daylight and color vision (10)

congestive heart failure   Abnormal condition in which blood flow backs ups and congests in lungs or extremities (11)

connective   One of the four principle types of body tissues; connective tissue is found in many body structures because it holds other tissues together or connects different types of tissues that make up the organs of the body (6)

constrict   Function in which the pupil of the eye gets smaller to restrict the amount of light that enters (10)

consumers   The customers of a particular business (1)

Contact isolation precautions   Used for patients known to be infected with a microorganism that is not easily treated with antibiotics and that can be transmitted easily between the patient and health care worker or from patient to patient (23)

continuous method   A method of liquid nutrition using a gastrostomy tube that involves a small amount of feeding continuously instilled in the PEG tube (26)

contraband   Restrictions in a health institution such as weapons, illegal drugs or alcohol, or smoking in a non-smoking area (17)

contractual basis   The basis in which workers are employed and given a fee for their services (2)

contractures   Abnormal shortening of muscle fibers; usually occur when individuals are immobilized for periods of time and when their limbs are not positioned in proper alignment (9)

contribution   Addition of information and service to the work of a team (17)

convex   One of the four normal curves of the spine; the thoracic, the sacral, and coccygeal areas are convex (curved outward) (8)

Cooley's anemia   Genetic disease in which deficient hemoglobin synthesis causes destruction and early breakdown of red blood cells (11)

cooperation   Contribution of a team member's best effort to accomplish team goals (17)

copulation   Term relating to the penis entering the vagina (15)

coronary arteries   The main vessels branching from the aorta supplying the heart muscle with blood (11)

coronary artery disease (CAD)   Any abnormality affecting the arteries of the heart (11)

corpora cavernosa   Vascular cave that becomes engorged with blood during sexual stimulation (15)

corpus callosum   Small bridge of tissue that connects the two hemispheres of the cerebrum (10)

corpus luteum   Developed from a follicle once ovulation occurs, it produces a hormone that readies the uterus for implantation of a fertilized ovum (15)

corticosterone   Adrenal cortex hormone that influences CHO, potassium, and sodium metabolism (16)

cortisol   Natural cortisone for the body produced by the adrenal cortex (16)

covert   Hidden; type of anger (20)

CPR (cardiopulmonary resuscitation)   A method of providing oxygen manually to vital organs following cardiac arrest until appropriate, definitive medical treatment can restore normal heart and pulmonary function (27)

cranial nerves   Twelve pairs of nerves that originate in the brain and send sensory messages to the brain or away from the brain (10)

creatinine   Normal alkaline constituent of urine (14)

critical pathway   A written document that outlines for the physician, nurse, and patient the expected or usual course of treatment for a specific DRG (1)

crutches   Devices used to assist in ambulation if an injury to the lower extremities has occurred, but upper-body strength remains intact (25)

culture   Mores of a people, which separates them from others (19)

Cushing's syndrome   results from a tumor of the adrenal cortex, or from a tumor of the pituitary gland, causing excessive secretion of ACTH (16)

cyanosis   Gray or bluish coloration of the skin (7)

cyclothymic disorder   Disorder characterized by depressed mood most of the day for a period of at least two years, but the severity of the symptoms are less severe and dysfunctional for the individual than a dysthymic disorder (21)

cystectomy   Removal of the bladder (14)

cystitis   Inflammation of the bladder (14)

cystoscope   Instrument inserted into the urethra to visually exam the bladder (14)

cytoplasm A jellylike substance outside the nucleus of a cell and within the cell's membrane (6)

daily weights Weights ordered for patients with edema (25)

data entry The entering of information into a special computer program (3)

death with dignity Concept that every person should have the right to die without pain and in a peaceful manner (20)

deciduous teeth Baby's full set of teeth, which are eventually replaced by secondary teeth (13)

decubiti A term used to refer to a breakdown of skin tissue that occurs when blood flow is interrupted (Also called pressure sores, bedsores, decubitus ulcers, or pressure ulcers.) (25)

decubitus ulcers Also called bedsores, pressure sores, or pressure ulcers; areas of skin breakdown (25)

decubitus ulcers Sores on the skin caused by pressure, especially from bony prominences (7)

defense mechanisms Coping strategies that include denial, projection, displacement, compensation, suppression, regression, and repression (21)

delegation Act of appointing certain tasks and duties to others (17)

delirium tremens (DT's) Seizures, severe agitation, confusion, and hallucinations caused by withdrawal from alcohol or other substance (21)

delirium The grossly abnormal impairments of mental functioning that result from a medical condition or a chemical- or substance-induced cognitive dysfunction (21)

delusion Belief that something is true when it isn't; a false belief that cannot be altered by relating the truth (21)

delusional disorder A disorder that appears to function within the normal limits in most life areas except for one irrational belief that cannot be shaken even when logical evidence supports its fallacy (21)

dementia Once referred to as senility, this state results from a degeneration of brain tissue and is chronic in nature with a slow onset, unlike delirium (21)

dendrites One of the three main parts to the neuron, which are short projections that protrude to form a treelike mass of short branches extending from the cell body and conduct messages to the cell body (10)

denial One of the five stages of death and dying; a coping mechanism in which the person does not believe reality (20)

dentures Artificial teeth (25)

dependence the need to use a substance (21)

dependent personality disorder Disorder that is characterized by submissive behavior, helplessness when alone, fear of abandonment, and the inability to make decisions (21)

depression An emotional state characterized by extreme feelings of dejection, worthlessness, hopelessness, and sadness (22)

depression One of the five stages of death and dying in which a person withdraws and expresses sadness (20)

depressive episodes Episodes that include at least five or more of the following symptoms: insomnia; hypersomnia; slowness of motor activity; feelings of worthlessness, uselessness, helplessness, hopelessness; recurrent thoughts of death and/or suicide; lack of concentration; feelings of guilt; weight loss or gain; and a lack of interest or pleasure for any activity (21)

dermis The second layer of skin that is composed of connective tissue (7)

descending colon Part of the colon that lies in the lower left abdominal cavity (13)

despair Part of the eighth stage in Erikson's developmental theory; to lose all hope of confidence (19)

development Physiological, psychological, and social growth to full size or maturity (19)

diabetes insipidus Diabetes that is caused by a deficiency of the antidiuretic hormone, ADH; produces excessive thirst from excessive urination (16)

diabetes mellitus "Sugar diabetes"; a disease that results from a lack of insulin production in the pancreas (13)

diagnostic related groups (DRGs) Groups of related or similar diagnoses that have a standardized length of hospital stay and standardized costs for treatments (1)

dialysis External means of compensating for loss of kidney function; performed by peritoneal dialysis or hemodialysis (14)

diaphoresis Profuse sweating (18)

diaphysis In long bones, the central shaft of the bone (8)

diastolic pressure Pressure that is always present in the blood vessels and is measured when the heart relaxes, written as the lower number of the blood pressure (25)

diffusion Passage of fluid from an area of greater concentration to less (14)

digestion The breakdown of food achieved both mechanically and chemically (18)

digestion The process by which food substances are broken down into absorbable nutrient molecules (13)

digestive system   The tract from the mouth to the anus including all the organs and glands associated with food digestion (13)

dilate   To make wider or larger; for example, when the pupil of the eye dilates, it allows more light to enter (10)

disgust   Marked aversion aroused by something highly distasteful; component of Erikson's eighth developmental stage (19)

diskette   A 3-1/2-inch plastic wafer cartridge that permits portable storage on a computer (3)

disorganized schizophrenia   Schizophrenia characterized by incoherence, grossly disorganized behavior, flat or inappropriate affect, fragmented delusions, stereotyped behavior with grimaces, mannerisms, and social withdrawal (21)

dissociative disorder   Also called multiple personality disorder, this evolves as a response to deep emotional and physical abuse and results in a lack of personality integration (21)

distorted thinking patterns   Patterns of thinking that involve judging self, others, and values with each one denying reality and trying to conform reality to one's beliefs, creating emotional turmoil (21)

diverticulitis   Inflammation of small distended sacs or outputchings called diverticula along the intestinal lining, especially the colon (13)

diverticulosis   "Condition of little diversions"; outpouchings along the colon wall due to weakened musculature (13)

DNA   Ladder of amino acids that form a genetic code (6)

dorsal lithotomy position   Position used for gynecological and urethral exams and procedures, in which the patient is supine with the knees flexed (25)

Down's syndrome   One of the genetic causes of mental retardation that results from trisomy of chromosome 21 (21)

droplet isolation precautions   Used for patients known or suspected to be infected with microorganisms transmitted by droplets during coughing, sneezing, talking or performance of procedures that induce coughing (23)

ductless glands   Glands that secrete substances directly into the blood rather than through a tube or duct into another organ (16)

ductus deferens   Duct that carries sperm from the epididymis to the common ejaculatory duct (15)

duodenum   The first of three sections of the small intestine (13)

Duoderm dressing   Wafer-type dressings that provide a protective "second skin" for wounds (26)

duoderm   Dressing that acts as a second skin; literally, "two-skin" (7)

durable power of attorney   A document that appoints a specific person to make treatment decisions for an individual when the patient is unable to make those decisions personally (20)

dwarfism   Result of an underproduction of growth hormone; frame is short but arms and legs are in normal proportion (16)

dysmenorrhea   Painful menstrual flow (15)

dysphagia   Difficulty swallowing (25)

dyspnea   Difficulty breathing (12)

dysrhythmias   Disturbances or abnormalities in the normal pattern of the heart (11)

dysthymic disorder   disorder that is characterized by depressed mood most of the day for a period of at least two years (21)

ECG paper   Specially coated paper that accommodates the stylus and mark of an ECG appropriately (26)

ectopic pregnancy   Abnormal pregnancy in which the embryo fails to migrate to the uterus to implant on the wall of the uterine lining (15)

eggcrate mattress   Foam mattress used to prevent decubitus ulcers (25)

electrocardiogram (ECG)   A record of the electrical activity of the heart which shows certain waves and gives important information concerning the spread of excitation to the different parts of the heart; it is of value in the diagnosis of cases of abnormal cardiac rhythm and myocardial damage (3)

electrolytes   Positive or negative charged salts necessary for various body functions (14)

electronic thermometer   Digital instrument used to measure temperature (25)

elimination   Excretion of wastes from the body (18)

elimination   Process of ridding the body of unusable solid waste products (13)

elimination   Removal of waste products, as in urine from the body (14)

emboli   Traveling blood clots (25)

embolus   Refers to a thrombus that circulates in the bloodstream until it becomes lodged in a vessel; such as a blood clot that travels to the brain (10)

embryonic disk   Organization of the layers of cells that will become the organs and systems of an embryo (15)

empathy   The ability to understand or experience another's situation, pain, or happiness, through that person's perspective, rather than one's own (24)

emphysema   Condition that results from chronic inflammatory and obstructive conditions of the bronchi and the lungs (12)

empty calories   Calories in foods that provide quick energy in the form of refined sugar and saturated fat, but they supply no vitamins or minerals (18)

end-result reinforcement   Strengthening of a desired behavior usually by reward of that behavior that is given once a task is entirely completed (22)

endocardium   The inner lining of the heart (11)

endocrine glands   Glands that have no ducts; their secretions are absorbed directly into the blood (6)

endometriosis   Abnormal gynecological condition that involves cells of the uterine lining growing in areas of the body other than the uterus (15)

endometrium   Inner layer of the uterus (15)

enema   Procedure for injecting fluid into the bowel through the anal orifice (25)

enteritis   Inflammation of the small intestine (13)

enterostomal therapist   A resource nurse who specializes in treating colostomy patients (13)

environment   All the surrounding conditions and influences affecting the life and development of an organism (23)

enzymes   Chemical substances that act as catalysts to produce a chemical reaction (13)

epidermis   The outer surface of the skin made up of several layers of epithelial tissue (7)

epididymis   Duct located at the upper end of each testis, which leads to the ductus deferens (15)

epiglottis   Cartilage shaped like a leaf, located on top of the thyroid; cartilage in the larynx that acts like a lid when it closes the entrance to the larynx during swallowing (12)

epilepsy   A disorder in which the primary symptom is seizure or convulsion (27)

epilepsy   Seizure disorder that may be caused by trauma or infections of the brain (10)

epinephrine (adrenalin)   hormone secreted by the adrenal medulla, critical to the body's response to stress; "flight or fight" hormone (16)

epinephrine   Hormone that stimulates or accelerates reactions; also called adrenaline (10)

epiphysis   Each end of the long bone (8)

epithelial   One of the four principle types of body tissues; epithelial tissue is designed to secrete and absorb substances (6)

erythrocytes   Red blood cells (11)

esophagitis   Inflammation of the esophagus (13)

esophagus   Food pipe, which is a muscular organ lined with a mucous membrane that connects the pharynx or throat with the stomach (13)

estrogen   Female hormone that helps the female to maintain her feminine characteristics and to continue reproductive functions (16)

ethical dilemma   Conflict regarding moral decisions concerning the treatment plan of the patient (20)

ethics committee   Committee that is consulted when ethical dilemmas arise in health care institutions (17)

ethics   Refers to a moral code and standards of conduct that guide the behavior of persons in a particular profession (17)

ethnicity   Groups of people within a cultural system who are given special status based on religion, language, or appearance (19)

etiology   The cause of a condition (8)

euphoria   A sense of well-being that is seen often in situations of addiction; the initial indulgence of it can spark a positive reinforcement for continued use of a substance (21)

evaluating   Step in the nursing process in which the nurse decides if a solution was successful in resolving a problem (17)

exacerbation   An increase in the seriousness of a disease or disorder, such as a particular "flare-up" of a certain system of the body (10)

expectorate   To dislodge mucous secretions adhering within the lungs (26)

expiration   Exhaling of air (12)

extension   One of the terms used to describe the normal range of motion of joints and muscles; the action that makes the angle of a joint larger (9)

external ear   One of the three main sections of the ear; the portion of the ear that is visible on the side of the head (10)

face mask   A type of oxygen delivery in which a mask is fitted over the nose and the mouth (26)

fallopian tubes   Uterine ducts that carry the ovum from the ovaries to the uterus (15)

fat-soluble   Vitamins that cannot be dissolved in water, but can be stored by the body (18)

fats   Substances made from carbon, hydrogen, and oxygen, they are a concentrated form of energy

fecoliths   Fecal stones or undigested particles that get trapped in the diverticula of the colon (13)

femoral pulse   Pulse assessed to determine the presence of blood flow to the lower extremities (25)

fetus   Unborn human developing in the uterus from a fertilized egg from the eighth week to the fortieth week of pregnancy (15)

fiber   The indigestible carbohydrate and carbohydrate-like components of food (18)

fimbriae   Finger-like projections that sweep the ovum from the ovaries into the ducts of the fallopian tubes (15)

first-degree burns   Superficial burns that involve injury to the epidermis only (7)

flagella   Hairlike extensions on certain microbes that provide spontaneous movement (6)

flat affect   An individual lacks emotional expression of any kind despite the environment (21)

flexion   Action that reduces the angle of a joint (9)

Foley   Another name for an indwelling catheter; a flexible rubber tube with openings and an inflatable balloon near the tip and two or three ports at the distal end (26)

follicle-stimulating hormone (FSH)   hormone produced by the anterior pituitary that stimulates the male and female gonads to mature and to produce their respective reproductive cells (16)

foot elevators   Bed devices used to eliminate pressure and promote alignment (25)

for-profit   Organizations who provide services for a profit (1)

force   Energy that when applied causes motion or changes speed (11)

foreskin   Also known as the prepuce, it is a layer of skin located at the end of the penis, usually removed after birth (15)

Fowler's   Position in which the head of the bed is elevated 25, 45, or 90 degrees (25)

fractional urines   Sugar and acetone found in the urine; called this because they are documented as the fraction S/A (25)

fractures   Broken bones (8)

French gauge   A measurement of a Foley catheter that reflects the width of lumen of the catheter (26)

frontal lobes   Located in the front of the cerebrum, beneath the forehead, these lobes are responsible for conscious and voluntary motor activities (10)

fundus   Bulging upper part of the uterus (15)

gait belt   Ambulation belt used in conjunction with assistive devices to steady the patient and help prevent falls (25)

gallbladder   Hollow sac that lies behind the liver and stores bile produced by the liver (13)

gastritis   Inflammation of the mucous membrane of the stomach (13)

gastrointestinal (GI) system   The digestive system (13)

gastrostomy tube (GT)   Tube used to place liquid nutrition or formula directly into the stomach to provide nutrition for the patient who is unable to eat or drink (26)

gastrostomy   Surgical procedure in which a new opening is made into the stomach (13)

gel-filled cushions   Sometimes called "fat pads"' cushions that simulate adipose tissue, reducing pressure when sitting (25)

gender   Sex of an individual; male or female (19)

general anxiety disorder   Disorder that is associated with unrealistic or excessive worry about life circumstances for at least six months (21)

generalized seizures   Those seizures in which all of the cerebrum is involved (27)

generative   Having the power or function of originating or producing; not self-focused; part of Erikson's seventh developmental stage (19)

genes   Contain the heritage of each organism passed on to individuals by their ancestors (6)

genetic code   Universal information system in living cells that determines the mapping of specified characteristics in offspring (6)

genetic material   Synonym for DNA (6)

gigantism   Result of an excess production of growth hormone; results in growth greater than 7 feet (16)

glass thermometer   A slender glass cylinder filled with mercury that expands when exposed to heat; used to measure temperature (25)

glioma   Tumor of the glial cells of the brain (10)

globulins   Broad category of simple proteins (11)

glomerulus   Cluster of capillaries in the nephron (14)

glucagon   Hormone produced by the pancreas involved in the metabolism of glucose from fats, proteins, and stored glycogen (13)

glucagon   Hormone that works to increase the amount of circulating glucose that is present in the blood (16)

glucometer   A bedside testing device used to check blood sugar levels (13)

glucose   Simple sugar found in certain foods; one of many abnormal constituents that may be found in urine (14)

goiter   Enlargement of the thyroid gland, which is a visible swelling in the neck (16)

gonads   Male sexual organ, which produces sperm (15)

gout   Also known as gouty arthritis, a form of arthritis that is caused by the deposit of uric acid crystals in and around the joint tissues, resulting in inflammation, pain, and swelling of the joints (8)

Graafian follicles   Microscopic sacs or follicles that are located on the inner surface of the ovaries, each of which contain an ovum, or egg (15)

grand mal   Most dramatic form of epileptic seizure (10)

grand mal   Type of seizure; "full-blown" seizure that progresses through four phases: aura, tonic, clonic, and sleep (27)

grandiose delusion   Delusion of ideas of grandeur (21)

Grave's disease   Exophthalmic goiter (16)

gravity   Property of possessing weight, force of the earth's gravitational attraction (23)

growth hormone (GH)   Hormone secreted by the anterior pituitary that accelerates the growth of the body (16)

growth   Physical changes of the human body throughout the life span (19)

hallucinations   False sensory perceptions or distortions of the senses in which person hears, sees, feels, tastes, or smells objects or persons that are not real (21)

handwashing Cleansing the hands with soap and warm water to reduce the transmission of germs (25)

hard drive A device that stores files within a computer (3)

health care A term used to describe institutions that treat persons who are ill, rather than persons who are well (1)

health maintenance organizations (HMOs) Third-party payer or insurance company who pays for a large percentage of hospital costs (1)

heart rhythm Pattern in which the heart beats (25)

heat applications Therapeutic ordered to relieve pain, increase circulation, relieve muscle spasms, and promote healing (25)

heel and elbow protectors Protectors that prevent friction against bed linens (25)

height Vertical distance from the heels to the top of the head (25)

Heimlich maneuver Maneuver used to dislodge from the trachea food or another object that is obstructing air flow to the lungs (12)

Heimlich maneuver Most notable intervention technique for removing a complete airway obstruction from a choking victim (27)

hematologist A doctor who specializes in blood cell diseases (3)

hematuria Blood in the urine (14)

hemiplegia Paralysis on either the right or the left side of the body; usually due to a stroke (9)

Hemoccult Test used to detect occult (hidden) blood in the digestive tract (25)

hemodialysis Lifesaving procedure in which blood is drawn from the body into a machine that removes the wastes then returns the purified blood (14)

hemoglobin Complex protein-iron compound of the RBC that carries oxygen to the cells (11)

hemophilia Hereditary bleeding disorder in which there is a deficiency of one of the blood's clotting factors (11)

hemoptysis Coughing up blood (12)

hemothorax Condition that affects the thoracic cavity and is the result of blood in the thorax (12)

heparin An anticoagulant found in the liver (13)

hepatitis Inflammation of the liver (13)

herniated intervertebral disc A swollen intervertebral disc that results from the protrusion of the nucleus pulposus found in the center of the disc (8)

high-density lipoproteins (HDLs) A type of circulating lipoproteins which is approximately 20-30% of the total blood cholesterol (18)

hilum a depression, as in the kidneys where the major blood vessels enter and exit (14)

histrionic personality disorder Disorder that is characterized by displays of melodramatic and attention-seeking behavior (21)

hives A skin condition that usually develops as the result of an allergic reaction to foods, medications, and products applied to the skin (7)

home care departments Departments in hospitals that provide discharge planning for patients who require transitions from hospital to the home or other facility (2)

hormones Chemical messengers of the body (16)

hormones Chemical messengers secreted by the endocrine glands (6)

hospice Care that can be delivered in a residential setting or at home that offers support to patients with terminal illness and to their families (20)

human chorionic gonadotropin (HCG) Hormone present in a woman's urine and blood, which confirms pregnancy (15)

hydrocephalus "Water in the head"; condition that occurs when there is obstruction of the circulation of the CSF (10)

hydrocortisone Corticosteroid hormone that is synthesized and secreted by the adrenal glands (16)

hymen Thin fold of mucous membrane that partially or completely covers the opening to the vagina (15)

hyoid The bone that is located below the pharynx (13)

hyperglycemic When blood sugar levels are higher than normal (13)

hyperparathyroidism Result of the overgrowth of the parathyroid gland (16)

hypersomnia Excessive sleep (21)

hypertension Elevated blood pressure exceeding 140/90 (11)

hyperthyroidism Overstimulation of the thyroid gland by the anterior pituitary hormone TSH (16)

hypertrophy Overdevelopment of muscles; results from overexercising (9)

hypervitaminosis The toxic state reached when fat-soluble vitamins are taken in very large quantities (18)

hypoglycemia When blood sugar levels drop or become very low (13)

hypoparathyroidism Result of the removal of too much parathyroid tissue in the surgical treatment of hyperthyroidism (16)

hypotension   Blood pressure lower than 90/60, causing insufficient oxygenation of tissues (11)

hypothalamus   Part of the brain responsible for unconscious and autonomic control, including controlling the functions of the pituitary gland (10)

hypothyroidism   Results from the removal or destruction of the thyroid gland (16)

identity   Distinguishing character or personality of an individual (19)

ileitis (enteritis)   An inflammatory disease of the small intestine, usually in the area of the ileum (13)

ileostomy   Created by opening the last part of the small intestine, the ileum, and forming a stoma of ileal tissue on the surface of the abdomen (26)

ileostomy   Surgical creation of a new opening into the ileum with the formation of a stoma or hole on the abdomen through which fecal excreta is discharged (13)

ileum   The final third of three sections of the small intestine (13)

immediate reinforcement   Strengthening of a behavior that is usually by reward of that behavior given to an individual after each step of a task (22)

impaction   Hardened stools trapped in the lower colon (25)

implementing   Step in the nursing process in which the nurse performs all actions of a plan in order to solve a problem (17)

incapacitated   A term used to describe a person who is unable to recognize, understand, or weigh the risks, benefits, and alternatives of a proposed treatment; a person cannot be considered incapacitated without sitting before a judge or mental health magistrate who makes the determination of competence (20)

incentive spirometry (IS)   Device that measures the volume of air inhaled by a patient (26)

incisal   Biting surface of the front teeth (25)

incompetent   A term used to describe a person who is unable to recognize, understand, or weigh the risks, benefits, and alternatives of a proposed treatment (20)

incomplete proteins   Those proteins that only contain some of the nine essential amino acids and some of the 13 others (dried beans and legumes, etc.) (18)

incus   One of the three bones of the middle ear, which strike each other in sequence allowing sound waves to enter the inner ear (10)

industry   State of working to achieve a goal (19)

indwelling catheter   A sterile tube that is left in the urinary bladder to continuously drain urine from the bladder (26)

inferior   Reference term to describe a structure located below another (6)

inferiority   Of low or lower degree or rank; component of Erikson's fourth developmental stage (19)

infusion pump   A pump used to deliver material into an artery or vein (26)

ingestion   The act of taking in food and fluid by the mouth (18)

initiate   To start certain activities (19)

inner ear   Part of the ear that houses microscopic receptors for hearing and balance (10)

insertion   Place of attachment, such as of a muscle to the bone it moves (9)

insomnia   Inability to stay or fall asleep (21)

inspiration   Inhaling of air (12)

insulin-dependent diabetes mellitus (IDDM)   Type of diabetes mellitus for which the patient requires insulin injections (16)

insulin   A hormone produced by the pancreas that is necessary in transporting glucose into cells (13)

insulin   Hormone that works to decrease the amount of circulating glucose that is present in the blood (16)

intake and output (I&O)   Term that refer to a method of evaluating fluid balance in the body (25)

integrity   Quality or state of being complete or undivided (19)

integumentary system   A system that is considered to be both an organ and a system; the skin is an integumentary system (7)

intelligence quotient (IQ)   Determined by standardized tests that are designed to measure an individual's performance of typical academic—math, reading, science—content on paper-and-pencil tests (21)

intermittent reinforcement   Strengthening of a desired behavior usually by reward of that behavior given after an individual completes every two or three steps of a task (22)

interneurons   Located only in the brain and spinal cord, these carry messages between the sensory and motor neurons (10)

intervertebral disc   The cushion between each vertebra of the spine that helps to absorb shock and prevent friction (8)

involuntary   Occurring without conscious control or direction; for example, involuntary muscle tissue moves and functions without the person thinking about how to move the muscle (9)

iris   Donut-shaped muscle that is the colored part of the eye (10)

irritable bowel syndrome A stress-related disorder in which the bowel lumen has areas of constriction (18)

islets of Langerhans Special cells in the pancreas that produce the hormones insulin and glucagon (16)

islets of Langerhans Special cells in the pancreas that produce glucagon and insulin (13)

isolation Method or technique of caring for persons who have communicable diseases (23)

isometric Muscular contraction that does not produce movement (9)

isotonic A muscular contraction that generates movement of muscles (9)

IVAC A method of tube feeding in which formula is poured into a plastic bag, similar to an IV bag with tubing attached; the tubing is then threaded through the pump, which controls the rate of infusion

Jacksonian seizures Seizures that involve one side of the body (27)

jaundice Condition characterized by yellowness of the skin, sclera, mucous membranes, and body fluid due to bile pigment deposits (13)

JCAHO (Joint Commission on Accreditation of Healthcare Organizations) A commission that must accredit hospitals in order for them to receive federal funds or Medicare (1)

JCAHO accreditation Official approval by the JCAHO to a health care facility that has conformed with established standards of care (1)

jejunum The second of three sections of the small intestine (13)

job postings A listing of jobs available within the health care system that are posted in local community hospital personnel departments (4)

JOBST stockings Brand name of stockings worn by patients to prevent post-operative circulatory complications, such as traveling blood clots (Also called therapeutic stockings or hose; antiembolism stockings or hose; surgical stockings or hose; TED hose or stockings.) (25)

joints Also called articulations, these are the unions of two or more bones (8)

justice The assumption that by the distribution of costs and benefits to the individual, family, and society, fairness and equity is achieved (17)

ketoacidosis An acid state caused by the byproducts of fat metabolism (13)

ketones The byproducts of fat metabolism (13)

keyboard A board that is linked to a computer on which typing is completed; it is similar to typewriter keys and has added function keys (3)

kidney stones Stones passed through urine, found when urine is strained and sediment remains (25)

kidneys Pair of bean-shaped urinary organs in the dorsal part of the abdomen, one on each side of the vertebral column (14)

knee-chest position Position that is used as an alternative to Sim's position, depending on the patient's mobility, in which the patient is resting body weight on forearms and knees on exam table (25)

kyphosis The abnormal curve of the thoracic vertebrae of the spine (8)

labia majora Larger folds of skin that make up the vulva (15)

labia minora Smaller folds of skin that lie between the labia majora (15)

labor The birth process (15)

large intestine (colon) Muscular tube 5 feet long that compacts solid waste products of digestion into feces (13)

larynx "Voice box"; organ of the respiratory system (12)

laser Acronym for light amplification by stimulated emission of radiation; a device that emits intense heat and power at close range (14)

lateral Pertaining to the side; farthest from the midline (6)

least restrictive alternative Choosing the least restrictive environment or situation in order to solve a problem by following a series of options; the concept that is employed to make decisions about living arrangements, classroom settings, vocational or job settings, or treatment measures (21)

leukemia White blood cell cancer; characterized by an abnormally high leukocyte count (11)

leukocytes White blood cells (11)

leukopenia Decrease in the number of white cells (11)

license A document that is awarded to an individual by the state board of examiners after successfully passing the examination(s) (3)

licensure The assumption that a person who holds the license is safe, has met certain educational requirements, and through examination has demonstrated competence to possess that particular license (17)

ligament A tough, fibrous band of connective tissue that connects one bone to another (8)

lingual Side of the tooth nearest the tongue (25)

liver Accessory organ vital to the process of digestion and absorption of nutrients; produces bile, stores excess glucose, and detoxifies the blood (13)

living will   A type of advanced directive dictating the exact life-sustaining or prolonging treatments that the individual wants if incompetent to make those decisions (20)

long-term care   Care in which persons treated in nursing homes, convalescent homes, and rehabilitation centers will remain in the facility for a long period of time (2)

lordosis   An exaggerated concave or anterior curve of the lumbar area of the spine (8)

low-density lipoproteins (LDLs)   Type of circulating lipoproteins that is approximately 60–70% of the total blood cholesterol (18)

lungs   Primary organs of the respiratory system that extend from the clavicles to the diaphragm and are responsible for the exchange of oxygen and carbon dioxide (12)

luteinizing hormone (LH)   Gonadotrophic hormone produced by the anterior pituitary that stimulates the growth and actions of the gonads (16)

lymph nodes   Small oval structures that filter lymph fluid and fight infection (11)

lymph vessels   Structures that carry lymph; surround intstines and absorb globules of fat from digested foods and deposit this fat in body tissues (11)

lymph   Thin fluid originating in organs and tissues traveling via lymph vessels and entering the bloodstream at neck veins. (11)

lymphatic system   Large networks of vessels and fluid that help to protect and maintain the internal fluid environment (11)

magnesium   Mineral necessary for muscle function; an electrolyte (14)

malignant   Cancerous (10)

malleus   One of the three bones of the middle ear, which strike each other in sequence allowing sound waves to enter the inner ear (10)

mania   An expansive, persistent, elevated, or irritable mood that lasts for at least one week (21)

Mantoux test   Intradermal skin test used to test individuals for tuberculosis (12)

market   The technique in which you sell your talents and abilities to gain employment (4)

master gland   Anterior pituitary gland that controls the growth and secretion of other endocrine glands (16)

mastication   Process by which the teeth tear, grind, and chew food (13)

Material Safety Data Sheets (MSDS)   Data provided by the manufacturer or distributor of hazardous materials giving comprehensive information about the product (27)

mechanical digestion   Digestion that involves the activities of chewing, swallowing, churning (or mixing), peristalsis, and defecation (13)

mechanical hydraulic lifts   Devices used to move patients who are unable to tolerate usual transfer techniques (25)

medial   Pertaining to the middle or midline (6)

mediastinum   Center of the thorax (12)

medical diagnosis   A classification for a disease or condition (1)

medulla oblongata   Bulb-shaped protrusion that sits just inside the cranium above the spinal cord, which contains reflex centers that control respiration, heart rate, and blood pressure (10)

melanin   A chemical that determines the color of a person's skin (7)

melena   Stools that are black and tarlike in nature resulting from an ulcer in the duodenum (13)

menarche   Female's first menstrual cycle (15)

menarche   The onset of menstruation (18)

meninges   Protective membranes that cover the spinal cord and brain (10)

meningitis   Inflammation of the meninges, often caused by an infection that begins with signs of a respiratory infection (10)

menopause   Cessation or pausing of menstruation at the end of childbearing years (15)

menorrhagia   Excessive bleeding at the time of menstruation (15)

menstruation (menses)   Shedding of the endometrium and blood flow from the uterus through the vagina (15)

Mental Health Law of 1979   The law that stimulated the closure of state mental hospital facilities in which inpatient treatment was found to be not productive or efficient in the treatment of persons with mental conditions (2)

mental health/mental retardation (MH/MR)   Refers to a type of community facility funded by the county, Medicaid, private insurance, or a managed care facility that treats patients with mental diagnoses (2)

mental retardation   Characterized by a significantly less-than-average IQ, which is present before the age of 18 years (21)

Mercury (Hg)   Liquid metal that expands when heated, used in a thermometer to measure temperature (25)

mercury sphygmomanometer   Blood pressure apparatus using a mercury column (25)

metabolism   Process of breaking down and building up foods in the body (13)

metastasis   Spread of cancer from site of origin to other sites in the body (10)

method of transmission   How microbes are transmaitted (23)

microorganisms   Living things unable to be seen without a microscope (14)

microorganisms   Small, living plant or animal not visible to the naked eye (23)

midbrain   Reflex center that rests on top of the pons and is responsible for hearing and eye movements (10)

middle ear   Part of the ear that consists of the tiny hollow structure in the temporal bone (10)

midline   The middle (23)

minerals   Inorganic (nonliving) elements that regulate fluid and assist in various body functions (18)

Minimum Data Set (MDS)   A standardized assessment in which OBRA assures that every nursing home resident throughout the country is assessed in the same areas (2)

miscellaneous hormones   Hormones that act locally at the site where they are made (16)

mitosis   Type of cell division in which each daughter cell contains the same number of chromosomes as the parent cell (6)

mitral valve prolapse   Protrusion of one or both cusps of the valve resulting in incomplete closure (11)

mitral   Pertaining to the heart valve between the left atrium and left ventricle (11)

mobility   Ability to move (25)

monitor   The visual screen that displays the work completed on a computer (3)

monosodium glutamate (MSG)   A preservative that contains high levels of sodium (18)

mood disorders   Also called affective disorders, these occur because feelings are affected by thoughts and are a reaction to mental stimuli (21)

motor   Neurons that carry messages away from the brain and spinal cord (10)

mouse   A handheld device linked to a computer that rolls on a hard surface and enables control of computer functions by finger clicks (3)

mouth care   Oral hygiene (25)

mouth   First organ of digestion; where food enters (13)

mucus   Thick fluid secreted by mucous membranes (14)

multichannel ECG machine   An instrument used to record the heart's electrical activity that is capable of recording all 12 views of the heart simultaneously and is the most common machine (26)

multiple sclerosis   Disease of the central nervous system that results from inflammation or loss of the myelin coating on multiple nerve fibers throughout the central nervous system (10)

multiskilled worker   The term used to describe the expanded role of unlicensed care providers; a generic term used to describe a variety of service staff and clinical staff position descriptions (3)

muscle tone   Normal state of tension of the muscles (9)

muscular   One of the four principle types of body tissues; muscular tissue is composed of special cells that are designed to contract or to pull together to produce movement (6)

myasthenia gravis   Neuromuscular disorder producing sporadic progressive weakness and fatigue of skeletal muscles caused by faulty chemical transmission at the myoneural junction (9)

myocardial infarction (MI)   Occlusion of a coronary area resulting in necrosis or tissue death of part of the heart muscle (11)

myocardial infarction   Commonly called a heart attack; death of cardiac muscle occurs as a result of partial or complete blockage of one or more of the coronary arteries (27)

myocardium   Cardiac muscle tissue, which is not voluntarily controlled (9)

myocardium   Muscular layer of the heart (11)

myometrium   Middle layer of the uterus (15)

myxedema   Disease that results from hypofunction of the thyroid gland (16)

narcissistic personality disorder   Disorder that is characterized by a grand sense of self-importance and lack of empathy for others (21)

nasal cannula   The most common and simplest way to deliver oxygen, in which a hollow tube with prongs attached is placed in the patient's nose, while the tubing is hooked behind the ears and the chin (26)

nasogastric tube   A tube inserted through the nose, pharynx, esophagus, and into the stomach used for liquid feedings (18)

negative feedback   Process of regulating the activity of an endocrine gland by directly or indirectly stopping or slowing its activity (16)

negative reinforcement   Strengthening of a positive behavior by withholding reward or punishment when the behavior is not the appropriate or desired behavior (22)

nephrectomy   Surgical removal of the kidney (14)

nephrons   Microscopic structural working units of the kidneys located in the cortex (14)

nervous   One of the four principle types of body tissues; nervous tissue is composed of nerve cells called neurons; designed to receive messages from the environment, to send messages to the brain, and to direct and control the reactions of the body (6)

network   A series of computers linked together to share information and programs (3)

networking   Meeting people in your field of practice (other care professionals) that can lead to a job offer or can provide you with future assistance (4)

neurochemical   Protein substance that sends a message (10)

neurologist   A physician who specializes in neurologic disorders (3)

neuron   Basic structure or unit of the nervous system; a nerve cell (10)

neurosis   An anxiety-based disorder leading to maladaptive use of defense mechanisms (21)

neutropenia   Decrease in the number of neutrophils, a type of white blood cell (11)

nihilistic delusion   Delusion of denying the existence of some part of the self (21)

non-insulin-dependent diabetes mellitus (NDDM)   Type of diabetes mellitus for which the patient does not require insulin injections (16)

nonmaleficence   The assumption that health care professionals do not act in a manner that is knowingly harmful to the patient (17)

nonprofit   Organizations that do not provide services for a profit (1)

nonverbal   Communications messages that include appearance, professional image, body language, eye contact, facial expressions, physical distance, and personal space between people (17)

norepinephrine (noradrenalin)   hormone secreted by the adrenal medulla, critical to the body's response to stress (16)

normal sinus rhythm (NSR)   A pattern of heart rhythm with the conduction system of the heart firing in the predicted sequence (26)

nose   Organ of the respiratory system that is the first organ of breathing; it filters, moistens, and warms air before it enters the lungs (12)

nosocomial   Pertaining to or originating in a health care facility such as a hospital (23)

nostrils   Right and left openings to the nose, divided by the septum (12)

Nuclear Regulatory Commission (NRC)   The commission that inspects hospitals to ensure that radiation and radioactive materials used in medical imaging departments and in the treatment of patients are safe for the patient and the employees (1)

nucleus pulposus   A pulpy, gelatinlike substance that makes up an intervertebral disc (8)

nucleus   The brain of the cell; directs all of the cellular activities (6)

nurse extenders   The forerunners of the multiskilled worker; in health care, the utilization of unlicensed care providers (nursing assistants/clinical care associates) (1)

nursing process   Method of problem solving used by health professionals (1)

nutrients   Water, carbohydrates, proteins, fats, vitamins, minerals, and fiber that provide specific body functions (18)

nutrition   A collective process of taking in food and using it for proper body function, including growth, repair, and maintenance (18)

objective data   Factual information, including descriptive and accurate observations, results, and measurements (17)

OBRA (Omnibus Budget Reconciliation Act)   The law that regulates the business practices and care activities of the long-term care industry (2)

obsession   A persistent and often unreasonable thought that preoccupies one's thought processes (22)

obsessive-compulsive personality disorder   Disorder that is characterized by excessive orderliness and preoccupation with perfectionism, and mental and interpersonal self-control (21)

occipital lobes   Located at the posterior base of the cerebrum, responsible for sight and the interpretation of vision (10)

occlusion   Blockage in a vessel (11)

occupied bed   Making a bed with the patient in the bed (25)

oil-retention enema   Disposable enema with oil used to soften hardened stools, as with an impaction. (25)

olfactory bulb   Bulb at the core of the cerebrum that accomplishes the sense of smell (10)

oliguria   Scanty or very small amounts of formed urine (14)

oncology   Term used to describe the care of the patient with cancer (3)

open bed   Bed made with the top sheets fanfolded to the foot of the bed (25)

oral suction Yankeur catheter   A plastic tube with a thick grip for easy use to withdraw secretions or fluids from an airway through oral suctioning (26)

oral thermometer   Glass thermometer with a long slender bulb and a blue tip (25)

orchidectomy   Removal of the testis (15)

organelles Structures that carry out digestive, respiratory, and circulatory functions (6)

organic wastes End results of the metabolism of all ingested proteins (14)

organism A life-form; a living being that is made of many structures that are dependent on one another (6)

organs Parts of the body, made from different tissue, that have a specific function (6)

orifices Opening in the body—mouth, nose, ears, anus, vagina (23)

origin Fixed, or stationary, end of a muscle attachment (9)

orthopedist A specialist who deals with skeletal diseases (3)

orthopnea Difficult breathing that requires an erect sitting position (12)

OSHA (Occupational Safety and Health Administration) An administration that surveys or visits hospitals to ensure that they comply with safety and health codes established by this branch of government (1)

osteoarthritis The form of arthritis that often occurs as a result of the aging process (8)

osteoporosis A condition that results from the loss of calcium from the bone, which makes the bones porous and brittle, and they then can be easily broken (8)

ostomy care Involves caring for a patient who has a surgical stoma (26)

ova and parasites (O&P) Test used to detect worms and their eggs within the digestive tract (25)

ovaries Female gonads that produce the female reproductive cells, or ova (eggs) (15)

overt Blatant; type of anger (20)

ovulation Term that describes the rupturing of the follicle and the release of an egg (15)

ovum Egg produced by the ovaries (15)

oxisensor A light-sensitive device used to measure the saturation of oxygen in the patient's circulating blood (26)

oxytocin Hormone produced by the posterior pituitary that operates to effect labor and delivery of a baby and to prevent postpartum hemorrhage (16)

pain scale Method measuring the intensity of pain; one being mild and 10 being severe (11)

palate Area of the mouth that, along with the jaw bones, frames the buccal cavity (13)

pancreas An exocrine and endocrine gland, which produces two hormones (glucagon and insulin) and which also releases digestive juices rich in enzymes into the duodenum (13)

pancreatitis Inflammation of the pancreas (13)

panic disorders Disorders that are characterized by an attack of acute anxiety and "fight or flight" physiology (21)

Pap test Routine screening test for the presence of abnormal cell growth in the cervix (15)

paralysis The loss of muscle function or the loss of sensation, or the loss of both muscle function and sensation; results from trauma, infection, or injury to the brain or spinal cord (9)

paranoid schizophrenia A type of schizophrenic disorder wherein there are delusions of persecution, grandiosity, jealousy, or hallucinations with persecutory or grandiose content (21)

paraplegia Paralysis in which a person is paralyzed from the waist down (9)

parasympathetic Division of the autonomic nervous system in which the nerves that control parasympathetic responses stimulate the body during normal conditions of life (10)

parietal lobes Located on the top sides of the cranium, these lobes are responsible for the sense of touch, including the perception and sensation of pain, pressure, and temperature (10)

Parkinson's disease Disease characterized by motor disturbances caused by the lack of the neurochemical, dopamine, in the body (10)

partial care Indicates that the patient can do things alone, with little or no help from the nurse. (25)

partial seizures Those seizures in which only part of the cerebrum is involved (27)

passive range-of-motion exercises Exercises that are performed by the nurse or clinical care associate when the patient is unable to do so (25)

passive-aggressive personality disorder Disorder that is characterized by appearing to be very submissive, but the unexpressed anger these persons internalize causes them to be aggressive in situations unrelated to the anger (21)

pathogens Disease-producing organism (23)

Patient Self-Determination Act An act passed in 1990 that sanctions the use of three documents (advanced directives, durable power of attorney for health care, living will) to have a person's wishes written and predetermined (20)

patients The primary consumers or customers of hospitals (1)

pedal pulse Pulse measured when the circulatory status of the feet is in question (25)

pelvic inflammatory disease(PID) Infection of the uterus, fallopian tubes, and ovaries usually caused by STDs (15)

penis   One of the external genitalia, or the visible reproductive organs of males (15)

peptic ulcers   Ulcers that involve the pyloric area of the stomach and generally include ulceration of the mucous membranes of the stomach and the duodenum (13)

percussion   A respiratory care procedure that is performed to loosen mucous secretions in the lungs by consistently and rhythmically moving cupped hands against the exterior chest wall overlying the lungs (26)

percutaneous endoscopic gastrostomy (PEG)   A puncture method in which a gastrostomy tube is inserted on the left side of the abdomen just below the ribs (26)

perforation   Occurs when an ulcer has eroded through the muscular layer and contents of the stomach and duodenum escape into the peritoneal cavity (13)

pericardium   Fibroserous sac around the heart (11)

peripheral nervous system (PNS)   Nervous system, which can be subdivided into the autonomic nervous system and the spinal nerves and the cranial nerves (10)

peristalsis   Stimulated by the autonomic nervous system, it is the contraction of smooth muscles that moves food through the digestive tract (13)

peritoneal dialysis   Process of removing wastes from the blood through the abdomen (14)

peritoneum   The membrane that lines the abdomen (13)

persecutory delusion   The delusion that someone or something is out to harm the person (21)

personality disorder   Results when distorted patterns of thinking interfere with a person's relationships, work, and social life (21)

petit mal   Small epileptic seizure that is sometimes unnoticeable (10)

petit mal   Type of seizure; small seizure whose symptoms may include staring, "fading out" for a few seconds, or rapid blinking of the eyelids (27)

phagocytes   White blood cells that digest microbes and cellular debris (11)

pharyngitis   Inflammation of the throat (13)

pharynx   Throat; organ of the respiratory system that is responsible for respiration and digestion (12)

pharynx   Tubelike structure made of muscle and lined with a mucous membrane, which serves as a passageway for food to enter the esophagus (13)

phlebitis   Inflammation of a vein (11)

phlebotomy   Literally meaning "opening into a vein," it involves puncturing a vein to obtain a venous blood sample for laboratory analysis (26)

phobia   An intense, irrational fear of a person, place, object, activity, or situation (21)

phosphate   Salt necessary for blood acid-base balance (14)

phosphorous   Inorganic salt present in normal urine (14)

physiatrist   A physician who specializes in physical rehab medicine (3)

physician assistant   A person who usually holds a bachelor's degree in a particular medical field and is licensed in the state to perform physical examinations and to work with the doctor to treat patients; this person is not a nurse (2)

physiological   Pertaining to the normal functions and processes of the human body; basic needs including oxygen, water, and food (19)

physiology   The study of the function of an organism (6)

pinna   Visible part of the external ear, which collects sound waves that move along the external ear canal to the eardrum (10)

Pitocin   A trademark for an oxytocin (16)

pituitary gland   Pea-sized gland located below the hypothalamus (16)

placenta   Nest of blood vessels in the uterus in which the zygote is implanted during pregnancy (15)

planning   Step in the nursing process in which the nurse decides specific actions that need to be taken to solve a problem (17)

plasma proteins   Proteins such as albumin or globulin present in the blood; when present in the urine, they are indicative of renal disease (14)

plasma   Liquid portion of the blood that contains water and the protein substances albumin and globulin (11)

platelets   Thrombocytes, or clotting cells (11)

pleura   Protective membrane of the thoracic cavity (12)

pleural   Pertaining to the membrane that lines the thorax and protects the respiratory organs (12)

pneumatic (intermittent) pressure stockings   Stockings used on post-operative patients to prevent the complication of deep vein thrombosis (26)

pneumonia (pneumonitis)   Inflammation of the lungs (12)

pneumothorax   Condition that affects the thoracic cavity and is the result of air in the thorax (12)

polycystic disease   Kidneys bearing many cysts (14)

polyps   Outgrowths of the intestinal tract (13)

pons   Located directly above the medulla, it serves as a relay station by sending messages from the medulla to higher centers of the brain (10)

portal of entry   A way for a microbe to enter the human body (23)

portal of exit   A way for a microbe to escape the human body (23)

positive reinforcement   Reinforcement of a behavior that is usually considered a reward and is given at different intervals of time (22)

post-operative (post-op or surgical) bed   Bed prepared for a patient recovering from surgery; after surgery (25)

posterior (dorsal)   Reference term to describe the back, dorsal, or behind (6)

posterior lobe   One of the two portions of the pituitary gland (16)

potassium   An important positive ion necessary in maintaining intracellular fluid (14)

PPD (Purified Protein Derivative)   Substance used in intradermal test for tuberculosis (12)

precordial   Six wires splitting off from the central cable of an ECG machine (26)

prefix   A word component that begins a word and changes the meaning of the word (5)

pregnancy   Nine-month period during which the growth and developmental period of human life takes place (15)

premature ventricular contractions (PVCs)   Dysrhythmia in which the ventricle contracts out of sequence from the normal heartbeat; this can be a lethal rhythm (26)

prepuce   Foreskin at the end of the penis, usually removed after birth (15)

presbyopia   Condition of the eye when the lens of the eye loses its elasticity, thus it can no longer accommodate enough to bring near objects into focus; literally means "old vision" (10)

pressure sores   Term used to refer to a breakdown of skin tissue that occurs when blood flow is interrupted (Also called decubiti, bedsores, decubitus ulcers, or pressure ulcers.) (25)

pressure ulcers   Term used to refer to a breakdown of skin tissue that occurs when blood flow is interrupted (Also called decubiti, bedsores, decubitus ulcers, or pressure sores.) (25)

primary amenorrhea   Term used to describe a girl of 16–17 years who has not reached her menarche (15)

primary care   One of the three levels of health care in which measures and interventions are aimed at preventing illness and maintaining wellness or a state of optimal health (1)

primary nursing model   A nursing model that is based upon the premise that a professional nurse provides all the care to assigned patients from the day of admission to the day of discharge (1)

prn   As needed/as necessary (2)

production   To form, as in the formation of urine (14)

progesterone   Female hormone that prepares the inner lining of the uterus for pregnancy, maintains the development of the placenta, prevents the ovaries from producing ova during pregnancy, and decreases the contractions of the uterus during pregnancy (16)

prolactin (lactogenic) hormone   hormone produced by the anterior pituitary that promotes breast tissue growth during pregnancy and lactation, or milk production, after birth (16)

prone position   Position in which patient is lying on abdomen; used for spinal exams and procedures (25)

prostaglandins   Local, tissue hormones (16)

prostate   One of the glands that produce seminal fluid, located under the bladder and surrounding the urethra at this juncture (15)

protein   Class of hormones made from amino acids (16)

proteins   Substances composed of hydrogen, carbon, oxygen, and nitrogen; necessary for rebuild and repair (18)

psoriasis   A chronic inflammatory disease that is not infectious or contagious (7)

psychoactive substances   Drugs used to affect the mental state (21)

psychomotor seizures   Seizures that are varied in the appearance of the seizure activity and are a result of temporal lobe malfunction (27)

psychosis   A disturbance of thought, mood, social behavior, and judgment (21)

pulmonary edema   Swelling of the lungs due to the accumulation of fluid in lung tissue (12)

pulmonary embolism   Results from a blood clot that is lodged in a pulmonary artery (12)

pulse oximetry   The use of light to measure the saturation of oxygen in the patient's circulating blood (26)

pulse points   Areas along the body where pulse can be felt (11)

pulse   Heart rate (11)

pulse   Wave of oxygenated blood sent through the arteries with each contraction of the heart (25)

pupil   Open area of the eye located within the iris (10)

pyelonephritis   Inflammation of the renal pelvis and kidney (14)

quad cane   Cane with a four-prong supportive base often used when a patient is weak or paralyzed on one side (25)

quadrants   Imaginary scoring of the abdomen into four circular areas (6)

quadriplegia   Paralysis in which all four limbs are paralyzed (9)

quality assurance   The measurement and improvement of the quality of care provided by hospitals and health care facilities (1)

radial artery   Artery in the forearms used to measure pulse (11)

radial pulse   Pulse located on the thumb side of the inner wrist (25)

random-access memory (RAM)   The memory to which you have access in a computer; the temporary workspace memory of a computer (3)

rape   Sexual intercourse with a woman by a man without her consent and chiefly by force or deception (19)

rate   Number or numeric ratio. (11)

reactive psychosis   A short-term psychotic episode that evolves from an emotional turmoil and produces a brief period of schizophrenic manifestations with a return to pre-illness state after days, weeks, or months (21)

read-only memory (ROM)   The permanent data saved as special programs that permit a computer to operate (3)

recipe combinations   "Ingredient combinations" of prefixes, root words, and suffixes that help you to determine the meaning of most medical terms (5)

rectal thermometer   Glass thermometer with a rounded bulb and a red tip (25)

rectum   Part of the colon that is about 7–8 inches long and terminates at the internal anal sphincter (13)

regression   Returning behaviorally to an early stage of development (19)

remission   Disappearance of symptoms, as in multiple sclerosis (10)

renal artery   Main artery from the abdominal aorta leading to the kidneys (14)

renal calculi   Stones that form in the kidney (14)

renal failure   Condition when the kidneys do not produce urine (14)

renal pelvis   The expanded superior end of the ureter shaped like a funnel (14)

renal tubules   Tubular extension of the Bowman's capsule (14)

renal vein   Main vein exiting from the kidneys (14)

reservoir   Where microbes are hosted (23)

residents   Individuals who live in nursing homes or in long-term care facilities (24)

residents   The title given to consumers of long-term care facilities (2)

residual schizophrenia   Schizophrenia that results as an aftereffect of previous behavior (21)

residual   Residual feeding refers to any tube feeding formula that remains in the stomach that may not be digested (26)

respect for autonomy   Assumption that it is of the utmost importance to act in accordance with the values and beliefs of the patient (17)

respiration   Breathing (12)

respirations   Process of taking in oxygen and exhaling carbon dioxide (25)

restraints   Devices once considered a protective measure for persons who could fall or potentially inflict injury to self and others, now strongly discouraged in health care facilities (24)

résumé   The brochure that lists your talents and abilities for an employer (4)

retina   Inner most layer of the eye which is very vascular (10)

retroperitoneal space   Space behind the serous membrane that covers some of the abdominal organs; this the space in which the kidneys are located (14)

Rh factor   Antigen substance present in the erythrocytes of most people (11)

rheumatoid arthritis   A systemic disease (affecting more than one body system) with widespread involvement of the connective tissues, causing inflammation of the joints and the membranes that surround them (8)

rhythm   One of the characteristics used to describe the pulse; refers to the regularity or irregularity of the heart's contraction (11)

ritual   Repetition of an act or acts (22)

rods   Specialized types of microscopic receptors that respond to light rays that enter the retina; they are sensitive to dim light and are needed for good night vision (10)

rugae   folds in the mucous membrane of an organ, such as the stomach (14)

rugae   Folds of mucous membrane that line the stomach, vagina, and urinary bladder (13)

rule out   R/O, eliminated (23)

sadistic personality disorder   Disorder that is manifested by cruel and very aggressive behavior without concern for others (21)

saline enema   Enema made with .9% NS, which is isotonic; mimics body fluid (25)

salpingectomy   Surgical removal of a fallopian tube (15)

saturated fat A source of cholesterol in food; it is solid at room temperature (18)

schizoaffective disorders Disorders that involve schizophrenic features along with coexisting manic or depressive symptoms (21)

schizoid personality disorder Disorder that is seen in persons who demonstrate indifference to the social arena and those who have restricted affect or expression of mood with the lack of ability to experience emotion (21)

schizophrenia Gross fragmentation of thought and great disorganization of behavior and judgment; split or fragmented mind (21)

schizotypal personality disorder Disorder that is displayed by defects in interpersonal relationships and oddities in appearance, thinking, and behavior (21)

sclera Layer of tough connective tissue called the white of the eye (10)

scoliosis The sideways curve of any section of the vertebrae of the spine (8)

scope of practice Framework of boundaries and expectations from which one is presumed to function (17)

scrotum Sac that hangs behind the penis, which holds the testes outside of the body (15)

second-degree burns Partial-thickness burns that involve injury to the dermis and are characterized by blisters on the surface (7)

secondary amenorrhea Expected lack of menstrual flow that occurs during pregnancy (15)

secondary care One of the three levels of health care in which measures and interventions are aimed at treating illnesses before they necessitate hospital treatment (1)

secondary teeth Set of teeth (approx. 28–32) found in the adult mouth (13)

security thermometer Thermometer used for axillary, oral, or rectal temperatures; has a bulb similar to that of a rectal thermometer but is marked the same as an oral thermometer; also know as a "stubby" thermometer (25)

seizure Condition in which there are electrical disturbances in the brain (27)

self-actualization A quest to find one's identity, the purpose of one's life and existence (19)

self-esteem internal value and worth recognized by oneself (19)

seminal vesicles One of the glands that produce seminal fluid (15)

seminiferous tubules Tubes that are coiled within each testis, which are responsible for the production of spermatozoa (15)

sensory Neurons that bring messages to the brain and spinal cord (10)

septic shock Shock caused by massive infection or adverse reaction to medications (27)

septum A vertical partition separating the right and left sides of the heart. (11)

septum Wall or partition that separates the right and left nostrils (12)

service associate Unlicensed assistant providing transport, housekeeping, and related duties (3)

sexuality Collective characteristics that make the differences between male and female (19)

shaping Molding a behavior or teaching the approximate steps of a behavior or task (22)

shock Most commonly associated with a decrease in the volume of blood, meaning insufficient blood circulation to all parts of the body (11)

shock Not a disease but a warning signal that the body is in grave danger; blood flow is redirected to the internal organs (27)

shunt Artificial connection such as the surgical connection of an artery and vein used for hemodialysis (14)

sickle-cell anemia Hereditary disorder in which the red blood cells develop abnormally in shape and therefore cannot carry oxygen (11)

sigmoid colon Segment of the colon that makes an s-shaped turn and connects to the rectum (13)

Simmond's disease Condition that results from the removal of the pituitary gland, from a lesion in the blood vessels of the pituitary, or from a tumor of the pituitary. The thyroid and adrenal glands are unable to function because the stimulating hormones are absent (16)

simple fracture A broken bone when the bone does not protrude through the skin (8)

Sims' position Left lateral position that is used for rectal exams and procedures (25)

single-channel ECG machine An instrument used to record the heart's electrical activity that records each of the 12 leads individually (26)

sinoatrial (SA) node The pacemaker of the heart (11)

sinuses Four pairs of cavities in the bones of the head and face (12)

sitz bath Procedure designed to soak the perineal area in water without immersing the patient in a full tub of water (25)

skeletal One of the three types of muscles; these mucles are attached to bones and move the bones of the body; skeletal muscles are made of fibers that have a striped appearance (9)

small intestine   Tube of smooth muscle that is approximately 15–20 feet long and lies coiled within the abdominal cavity (13)

smooth visceral   Muscle tissue that works involuntarily, has a smooth, nonstriated appearance, and is found in the digestive organs, blood vessels, the skin, and some of the organs of the urinary system (9)

soapsuds enema (SSE)   Manually prepared soap and water solution (usually 500 to 1,000 cc) used to irrigate and cleanse the colon (25)

sodium   electrolyte; a positive ion necessary for cell integrity (14)

specific gravity   Test to determine the concentration of water in the urine (14)

sperm   Male seeds of reproduction (see spermatozoa) (15)

spermatozoa   Male seeds of reproduction; each microscopic sperm is a single cell with a head, neck, and tail (see sperm) (15)

sphincter   Round muscle that opens and closes (13)

sphygmomanometer   Apparatus used to measure blood pressure (11)

sphygmomanometer   Instrument used for measuring blood pressure (25)

spinal nerves   Thirty-one pairs of nerves that enter and exit all along the spinal cord, which are involved in sensation and movement of the arms and legs and connect with nerves of the central nervous system and the autonomic nervous system (10)

spleen   Organ of the lymphatic system whose functions include defense, blood storage, and the destruction of red blood cells and platelets (11)

sputum   Mucus from the lungs (25)

stagnation   To become or to remain without flow or movement (19)

Standard precautions   Recommendations that must be followed to prevent transmission of pathogenic organisms by way of blood and body fluids (23)

stapes   One of the three bones of the middle ear, which strike each other in sequence allowing sound waves to enter the inner ear (10)

STAT   Term meaning that immediate action is necessary (16)

status epilepticus   Condition of continuous seizure activity (10)

sterility   Infertility, in which the cause cannot be remedied (15)

steroids   Class of hormones made from cholesterol (16)

stimulus   The cause of a behavior (22)

stoma   Artificial opening (14)

stoma   Artificially created opening or hole (12)

stomach   Strong muscular organ that lies in the upper left abdominal cavity just below the diaphragm (13)

stomatitis   Inflammation of the mouth (13)

straight catheterization   Insertion of a sterile tube into the urinary bladder performed to remove urine remaining in the bladder after voiding, to intermittently empty the bladder when a person is unable to void voluntarily, and to obtain a sterile urine specimen (26)

striated branching   Type of muscle tissue found in the heart; called "striated" because it has the striped appearance of skeletal muscle; called "branching" because the muscle fibers overlap and branch around one another, making the muscle tissue more durable and strong (9)

striated   Skeletal muscle that is made of fibers that have a striped appearance; they are attached to bone and move the bones of the body (9)

stroke   Occurs when a hemorrhage or blood clots form in a blood vessel in the brain or when a clot travels to the brain causing tissue death; also called cerebral vascular accident (CVA) (10)

stylus   Part of the ECG, which is the pen-tipped point that transcribes thermally the electrical message transmitted from the heart (26)

substance abuse   Another name for substance dependence (21)

substance dependence   Maladaptive pattern of substance abuse that leads to a clinically significant problem or impairment based on at least three or more of the following conditions: tolerance; withdrawal symptoms when the substance is not taken; long-term use of a substance; persistent desire for the substance; great deal of time spent obtaining the substance; lack of activity attendance because of the use of the substance; and use of a substance in spite of the knowledge that it may be detrimental (21)

suctioning   The process of withdrawing secretions or fluids from an airway with a catheter (26)

suffix   A word component that ends a word and changes the meaning of the word (5)

sugar and acetone (S&A)   Substances that should not be present in normal urine (25)

suicidal ideation   Expressed when an individual is contemplating the idea of suicide (22)

sulfate   Inorganic salt present in normal urine (14)

superior   Reference term to describe higher than, or situated above (6)

supine position   Horizontal recumbent position in which patient is lying flat on back; may be used for abdominal exams and procedures (25)

suprapubic cystostomy   Surgical procedure performed to create a new opening above the pubic bone for the removal of urine (14)

suprarenal   Another name for the adrenal glands (16)

Surgical stockings   Stockings used to prevent post-operative circulatory complications, thus the name surgical stockings (Also called therapeutic stockings or hose; antiembolism stockings or hose; TED hose or stockings; JOBST hose or stockings.) (25)

surrogate decision maker   A person who acts on behalf of the individual who is unable to make decisions because of permanent unconsciousness or incapacitation (20)

susceptible host   Person who is able to get a disease (23)

sympathetic   Division of the autonomic nervous system, called the "fight or flight" division because it readies the internal organs and muscles for stressful situations (10)

synapse   Juncture between two neurons where a signal is passed on from one neuron to the next (10)

system   A group of organs that act together to produce specific functions of the body (6)

systolic pressure   Vessel pressure, which increases when the heart contracts, written as the top number of the blood pressure (25)

tachycardia   Abnormally fast heart rate, greater than 100 beats per minute (11)

tachycardia   Rapid heart rate (12)

tachypnea   Rapid breathing (12)

task analysis   Breaking down a procedure into its simplest steps (22)

team nursing models   Those models that utilize LPNs and nursing assistants to deliver nursing care tasks with the RN serving as team leader (1)

teamwork   Each member of a team contributes equally input or contribution in the provision of continuity of care (17)

TED hose   Stockings used to prevent post-operative circulatory complications (Also called therapeutic stockings or hose; antiembolism stockings or hose; surgical hose or stockings; JOBST hose or stockings.) (25)

Tegaderm dressing   A clear adhesive shield that protects a wound from water and potential irritants (26)

telemetry technicians   Technicians whose job is to continuously observe the cardiac activity of patients attached to cardiac monitors (26)

telemetry   Monitoring heart rate by remote (11)

Temperature   Measurements of the balance of heat loss or heat gain in the body (25)

temporal lobe epilepsy   Epilepsy in which seizures occur that result from temporal lobe malfunction (27)

temporal lobes   Located at the lower sides of the cerebrum, around the area of the ears, these lobes are responsible for hearing and the interpretation of sound and spoken language (10)

tendons   Nonelastic cords that attach muscles to bones (9)

tertiary care   One of the three levels of health care in which measures and interventions are implemented if someone is admitted to a hospital for treatment (1)

testes   Pair of male gonads that produce sperm (see testicles) (15)

testicles   Pair of male gonads that produce sperm (see testes) (15)

testicles   the male gonads**testosterone**   Male hormone responsible for maintaining male characteristics (15)

tetany   Hyperactivity of the muscles (16)

thalamus   Relay center for sensory information that is being sent to the brain (10)

therapeutic diets   Prescription diets, modified in some way to improve certain health problems (18)

thermal thermometer   Heat-activated thermometer (25)

third-degree burns   Full-thickness burns that involve injury of the epidermis, dermis, and underlying tissues, with complete destruction of all layers of the skin (7)

thoracic   Pertaining to the chest cavity, which is subdivided into the right and left pleural cavities (12)

three-way Foley catheter   A catheter used for continuous irrigation and drainage of the bladder (26)

thrombocytes   Clotting cells; platelets (11)

thrombocytopenia   Abnormal decrease in the number of clotting cells (11)

thrombophlebitis   Inflammation of a vein causing a blood clot (11)

thrombus   Blood clot that forms in a blood vessel in the brain (10)

thymus gland   Primary central gland of the lymphatic system responsible for the development of T-cells; shrinks with age (11)

thyroid-stimulating hormone (TSH)   Secreted by the anterior pituitary that controls the growth and hormone production of the thyroid gland (16)

thyroxin (T4)   Thyroid gland hormone (16)

tissue   Group of similar cells that act together to perform a particular function (6)

tolerance   A need for increased amounts of a substance to achieve intoxication or the desired effect (21)

tongue   A skeletal muscle that lies on the floor of the mouth (13)

tonsils   Rounded mass of lymphoid tissue located in the pharynx (11)

total parenteral nutrition (TPN)   Hyperalimentation; solutions containing high levels of dextrose (26)

total parenteral nutrition (TPN)   Provision of the total calories needed by intravenous route for a patient who is unable to take food orally (18)

trachea   Windpipe; organ of the respiratory system that functions as a passageway for air to and from the lungs (12)

tracheostomy   Creation of a stoma and the placement of a tracheal tube to allow air to enter the respiratory system (12)

transient ischemic attack (TIA)   Mini-stroke that occurs when blood flow is hampered for a brief period of time and mild strokelike symptoms are noted (10)

transverse colon   Part of the colon between the ascending and descending colons (13)

trauma   Injury to the body (27)

triage   Screening and classification of sick, wounded, or injured persons during disasters to determine priority needs for efficient use of medical personnel, equipment, and facilities (27)

tricuspid valve   Three-point valve located between the right atrium and the right ventricle (11)

triiodothyronine (T3)   Thyroid gland hormone (16)

tube feedings   Liquid feedings that are administered through a nasogastric tube (18)

tuberculosis (TB)   Infectious disease of the lungs caused by the bacteria tubercle bacillus (12)

turgor   Elasticity of the skin (25)

tympanic membrane   Eardrum, which separates the external and the middle ear (10)

tympanic thermometer   Electronic device inserted into the external ear canal to measure body temperature (25)

ulcerative colitis   Inflammatory and ulcerative disease of the colon (13)

undifferentiated schizophrenia   A type of schizophrenic disorder characterized by delusions, incoherence, or grossly disorganized behavior. (21)

unlicensed   Without a license; refers to those individuals, or care providers, who do not attend a prescribed academic and clinical education program and do not take an examination that will award a license to practice (3)

unoccupied bed   Making a bed without the patient in it (25)

unsaturated fat   Fat that is not solid at room temperature and can be further divided into plant fats (18)

urea   Chief constituent of urine (14)

ureter   Long, narrow tube extending from the kidney to the bladder (14)

ureterostomy   Surgical creation of a new opening in the ureter for urine to be excreted (14)

urethra   Passageway from the bladder for the release of urine from the body (14)

urethral orifice   Opening to the urethra, located above the vagina, through which urine passes (15)

uric acid   One of the two waste products of protein metabolism; specifically, the end product of purine metabolism (14)

urinalysis   Analysis of the urine to detect any abnormalities in pH, color, or constituents (14)

urine dipstick   Reagent stick that is placed into urine to test for sugar content or other abnormalities (25)

urine   Fluid formed in the kidneys, stored in the bladder, and discharged through the urethra (14)

urinometer   Device for determining specific gravity of urine; also called urometer (26)

urometer   Device for determining specific gravity of urine; also called urinometer (26)

urosepsis   Infection in the bloodstream due to the buildup of waste products when the kidneys fail (14)

urostomy   An opening created for the passage of urine (26)

V leads   Precordial leads; the six wires splitting off from the central cable of an ECG machine (26)

vaginal orifice   Opening of the vagina (15)

valvular diseases   Acquired or congenital disorders affecting the valves of the heart (11)

vas deferens   Also known as the ductus deferens, it is the duct that carries sperm from the epididymis to the common ejaculatory duct (15)

vein   Vessel that carries blood to the heart (11)

venules   Small veins (11)

verbal   Messages communicated in spoken language and voice tone (17)

very low-density lipoproteins (VLDLs)   A type of circulating lipoproteins that is approximately 10–15% of the total blood cholesterol (18)

villi   Tiny fingerlike microscopic structures found within the mucous lining of the small intestine (13)

visiting nurses association (VNA)   A community-run organization that delivers health care services for all segments of the health care continuum (2)

vital signs (VS)   Determinations that provide information about body conditions, including temperature, pulse, respirations, and blood pressure (25)

vitamins   Organic compounds that assist in the regulation of certain body processes, including the building of tissue (18)

vocal cords   Two fibrous bands located in the larynx; when exhaled air passes through these cords, speech is accomplished (12)

voluntary   Striated muscle tissue used by an individual to control the movement of the skeleton (9)

vulva   Collective name for the female external genitals (15)

walker   Assistive device used for the ambulation of patients who have full upper-body functioning, but whose legs are weak and unsteady (25)

wander guards   Alarms located on the exit doors of long-term care facilities that sound when the doors are opened (to prevent residents from injury due to wandering off the grounds of the facility) (24)

water or alternating air mattress   A mattress that inflates and deflates to prevent pressure on the patient's skin (25)

water-soluble   Vitamins that can be dissolved in water, but cannot be stored in the body (18)

waxy flexibility   State in which someone's limbs will remain in a certain position until you move them again (21)

weight   An important assessment tool for determining fluid and nutritional status (25)

wellness   State of optimal health (2)

wet-to-dry dressing   Dressing that is used to promote healing in which the inner gauze when dried, removes the unhealthy tissue (26)

withdrawal   Complete and immediate removal of a drug on which a person is dependent, which can often lead to seizures, severe agitation, confusion, and hallucinations

womb   Uterus; a pear-shaped organ composed of a thick muscular wall and lined with a mucous membrane. It is responsible for the functions of menstruation, pregnancy, and labor (15)

word building   The process of building medical terms through combining various prefixes, root words, and suffixes (5)

word root   The foundation, or major, word component (5)

zygote   Fertilized egg (15)